Biomechanics Of Musculoskeletal Injury

Biomechanics Of Musculoskeletal Injury

Eric R. Gozna, M.D., F.R.C.S. (C)

Research Associate, Bioengineering Institute
University of New Brunswick, Active Staff
Dr. Everett Chalmers Hospital, Orthopaedic Surgeon
Fredericton Medical Clinic, Fredericton, New Brunswick

Ian J. Harrington, M.D., F.R.C.S. (C)

Assistant Professor, Department of Orthopaedic Surgery
University of Toronto, Toronto, Ontario, Canada

with special contribution by

Dennis C. Evans, M.D., F.R.C.S. (C)

Lecturer, Department of Orthopaedic Surgery
University of Toronto, Toronto, Ontario, Canada

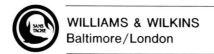

WILLIAMS & WILKINS
Baltimore/London

Library of Congress Cataloging in Publication Data

Gozna, Eric R
    Biomechanics of musculoskeletal injury.

    Includes index.
    1. Musculoskeletal system--Wounds and injuries. 2. Fractures. 3. Human mechanics. I. Harrington, Ian J., joint author. II. Evans, Dennis C., joint author. III. Title.
[DNLM: 1. Biomechanics. 2. Musculoskeletal system--Injuries. WE100 G725b]
RD680.G65   617'.47   80-16573   ISBN 0-683-03728-5

Composed and printed at the
Waverly Press, Inc.
Mt. Royal and Guilford Aves.
Baltimore, Md. 21202, U.S.A.

Dedication

To our Wives and Children

Preface

Virtually all of the members of the Orthopaedic Faculty at the University of Toronto have contributed in some way to this text, as most of the concepts are those which were transmitted through rounds, seminars, or informal discussions at the various teaching hospitals. Under the leadership of Professor Robert B. Salter, the basic philosophy of orthopaedic training at the University of Toronto has been that important concepts must be conveyed in a systematic and simplistic manner. We hope this textbook complies with that basic philosophy.

It was to Professor Donald R. Wilson that we originally presented the idea of a biomechanics textbook written by two orthopaedic surgeons who were originally trained as professional engineers. Had it not been for his encouragement and support, it is unlikely that the present book would have become a reality. Doctor Wilson continues to be an inspiration to those surgeons who have trained under him.

Dr. Dennis Evans's chapter on spinal injuries represents a career-long interest in this subject. This dates to his involvement in the Spinal Injuries Unit in Manchester, England, where he worked with Doctor Holdsworth. We are grateful to Dr. Evans for contributing this valuable chapter to our text; no engineer could have done it with greater clarity and few surgeons with a greater wealth of experience.

Miss Margot Mackay, B.Sc., A.A.M., the Department of Art as Applied to Medicine, University of Toronto, has been primarily responsible for the illustrations in this text. She is a very talented artist who has the ability to convey complex concepts using illustrations that are elegant in their simplicity. Miss Mackay was assisted by Mr. Frederick Lammerich.

We wish to thank Ms. Barbara Tansill and the staff at Williams & Wilkins for the excellent job they have done in preparing this text. We also wish to thank Drs. John, Godin, Moriarity and the editorial staff of MediEdit, Toronto, as well as the Department of Photography of Toronto East General and Orthopaedic Hospital for their valuable contribution to this text.

EG

IH

Contents

CHAPTER 1

Biomechanics of Long Bone Injuries

Eric R. Gozna

It is essential for the orthopedic surgeon to have a clear understanding of the biomechanics of long bone injuries, as these are the most common major injuries that he will be required to treat. Following careful clinical assessment of the patient, the accurate interpretation of the radiographic fracture pattern is the single most important step in planning a treatment protocol.

Though most musculoskeletal injuries occur in a predictable manner, as dictated by the forces involved and the structure of the region, there are always certain fractures that are unique to each injury. These fractures constitute the "personality" of that injury and distinguish it from all others. The purpose of this chapter is to describe a few of the underlying biomechanical principles that contribute to the unique characteristics of long bone injuries and to describe a systematic biomechanical approach for anticipating any long bone fracture pattern.

When confronted with the radiographs of a long bone fracture, the surgeon should remember the five factors responsible for any bony injury, three of which depend upon the characteristics of the *load* and two upon the characteristics of the *bone*:

Load characteristics
1. Type of load
2. Magnitude of load
3. Load rate

Bone characteristics
1. Material properties of bone
2. Structural properties of bone

Through systematic analysis of the radiographs and individual consideration of these factors, the surgeon can derive a great deal of information about the injury, such as the type of load involved, the amount of energy expended, the location of remaining soft tissue and periosteal hinges, and an estimate of the degree of associated soft tissue injury (anticipating

1

Table 1.1. Fracture Patterns Resulting from Combinations of Compression, Bending, Torsion

Fracture Pattern	Load	Appearance	Common Sites
Diaphyseal impaction	Axial compression		Intercondylar humerus, femur, tibial plafond
Transverse	Bending		Any long bone diaphysis
Spiral	Torsion		Any long bone diaphysis; frequently tibia, humerus
Oblique transverse (or butter-fly)	Axial compression + bending		Femur, tibia, humerus
Oblique	Axial compression + bending + torsion		Tibial-fibular, forearm

potential complications). In this manner the surgeon can fully define the personality of the particular injury.

The following sections will describe in detail the five factors listed above and the role that they play in the biomechanics of long bone fractures.

TYPE OF LOAD

Engineers refer to the application of a force to an object as *loading*. An object can be loaded in four ways: tension (traction or pulling apart), compression (pressing together), bending (angulation), and torsion (twisting). In medieval times the rack provided an ideal experimental model for pure traction injuries. As history books will attest, the major injuries resulting from this form of torture were to joints and ligaments and not to long bones. Hence, pure tension loading rarely produces injury to long bones. The clinically important ways in which long bones can be loaded are therefore combinations of compression, bending, and torsion. Table 1.1 summarizes the types of fractures which result from the various combinations of loads. The five basic injury patterns which result from combinations of compression, bending, and torsional loads are: diaphyseal impaction, transverse, oblique transverse, spiral, and oblique fractures.

Diaphyseal Impaction Fractures

If a short cylinder of homogeneous material is subjected to a compressive load applied through its center (i.e., axially), the fracture will propagate at an angle of approximately 45° with the center line, because this is the angle along which maximum stresses develop.[2, 8] Theoretically the material would fail along this plane, producing an oblique fracture pattern. In practice, however, it is difficult to apply a compressive load exactly through the middle of a cylinder, and, as a result, one portion is subjected to greater compressive loads than others.[11] If a cylinder is long enough, e.g., a human long bone, bending movements are created and a phenomenon known as "column buckling" occurs. In this response, the material tends to bend and collapse rather than to sheer at an oblique angle.

Fortunately, in dealing with long bone compression fractures, the orthopedist rarely needs to consider column buckling or pure oblique fracture configurations because, in long bones, an axially applied load

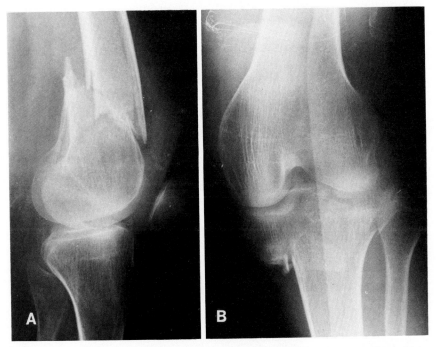

Figure 1.1. Two examples of diaphyseal impaction fractures resulting from longitudinal compression loads are the "Y" type supracondylar fracture of the femur (*A*) and the comminuted tibial plateau fracture (*B*).

usually drives the diaphyseal bone, with its thick rigid cortex, into the thin metaphyseal bone like a battering ram.[16] The resultant diaphyseal impaction fraction is the most common fracture pattern stemming from axial loading of long bone. Examples of this fracture pattern are supracondylar femoral fractures (Fig. 1.1*A*), tibial "plafond" and comminuted tibial plateau fractures (Fig. 1.1*B*).

Transverse Fractures

A bending load applied to a long bone subjects that portion of the cortex on the concavity of the bone to compression forces while it subjects that on the convexity to tension forces (Fig. 1.2). Cortical bone is weaker in tension than in compression[2, 3, 11, 13]; hence, it generally will fail in tension before it fails in compression. The crack begins on the tensile side of the cortex, and when the outer layers of bone fail, the layers immediately under this are subjected to maximum stress and fail. As successive layers fail, the crack propagates at right angles to the long axis of the cylinder and produces a transverse fracture line.

As half of the cylinder is under compression and the other half is under tension, there is a point between these two regions ("the neutral axis")

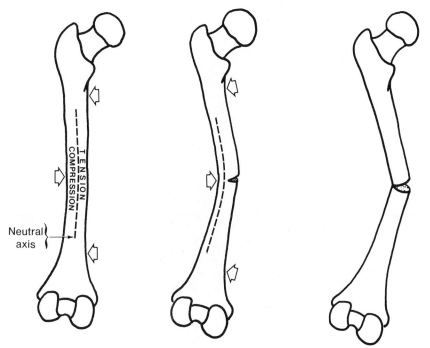

Figure 1.2.   Transverse fracture—bending load.

where there are no tension or compression forces. As the crack propagates across the bone, the neutral axis moves from the midline towards the cortex on the concave side of the bone (Fig. 1.2).

Oblique Transverse and Butterfly Fractures

These fracture patterns result from a combination of axial compression and bending (Fig. 1.3). As described earlier, pure axial loading should produce a uniform compression force throughout the bone, whereas bending produces compression forces on one side and tension forces on the other. When these two loads are combined, the net effect is to add to the compressive forces on the concavity and to subtract from the tension forces on the convexity. As a result of the combined axial compression and bending loads, several modes of failure can occur.

1. If the compressive forces are sufficiently large relative to the bending forces, the bone fails in compression, producing an oblique fracture.

2. If, on the other hand, the bending forces are sufficiently large, the stress will produce a pure transverse fracture.

3. Most commonly a combination of the two produces an injury known clinically as the oblique transverse fracture.[2] As the name implies, this fracture pattern is partially oblique (representing failure in compression) and partially transverse (tension failure).

Radiologically this pattern looks like a transverse fracture with one fragment containing a protuberance or "beak" (representing the oblique component).

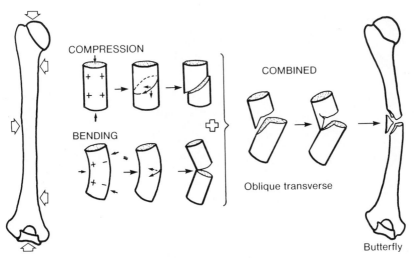

Figure 1.3. Butterfly and oblique transverse fractures—combined axial compression plus bending loads.

The butterfly fracture is a variation of the oblique transverse pattern. As the fragments continue to angulate, owing to the bending load, the fragment containing the oblique segment (beak) is impacted against the other fragment. Consequently the beak is sheared off, producing the classical butterfly fracture (Fig. 1.3).

Oblique transverse and butterfly fractures are commonly seen in the lower extremities when the thigh or calf receives a lateral blow during weight bearing; this fracture is common among pedestrians injured by automobiles (Fig. 1.4).

Spiral Fractures

There is controversy as to whether bone, when subjected to torsional loads, fails as a result of shearing—one portion sliding over another—or tension—pulling apart of intermolecular bonds.[3, 4, 13, 27] In any event, the

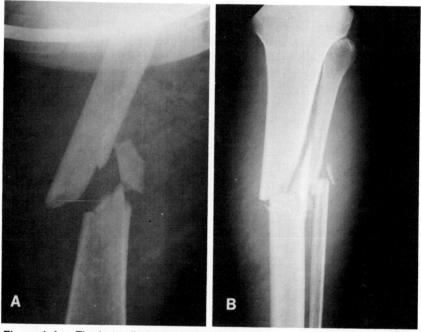

Figure 1.4.   The butterfly fragment is always located on the compression side of the bone. These x-rays are from pedestrian accidents and give a great deal of information about the mechanism of injury. The x-ray on the left (*A*) shows a femoral fracture resulting from a direct blow to the lateral side of the thigh by the bumper of a transport truck. The butterfly fragment is located on the lateral (compression) side of the femur. The radiograph on the right (*B*) is that of another patient struck on the anterolateral aspect of the calf by a sports car. As would be anticipated, the butterfly fragment is situated anterolaterally.

resulting fracture takes the form of a spiral propagating around the shaft at an angle of 40–45° with the long axes of the bone.[3, 4, 27, 28]

The mechanics of a torsional spiral fracture can be illustrated by drawing a square on the side of a rubber tubing (such as an operating room suction hose) and then twisting the tube. The square then changes to a rectangle, a change which implies that the long sides of the rectangle are under tension (i.e., stretched) and the other sides are compressed. If, as experimental data indicate,[2, 3, 4, 11, 13] adult cortical bone usually fails in tension before compression, the crack should propagate at right angles to the long sides of the rectangle (that portion under tension). Hence, the spiral should curve around the shaft in a direction that would allow the portion of bone under tension to open up. This is what happens. The spiral usually continues until the proximal and distal cracks are approximately one above the other and then a longitudinal crack appears to

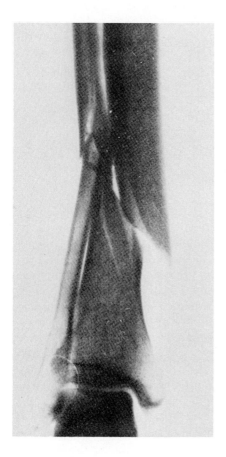

Figure 1.5.   Spiral fracture as the result of skiing injury. The ski tip caught in the snow, producing external rotation force through the calf. The direction of the spiral tibial fracture is that which would be expected from the history of the injury.

join these two points, producing the vertical segment of the spiral fragment.

The direction of the spiral indicates the direction of the torsional force producing the fracture. Figure 1.5 shows a spiral fracture of the tibia resulting from an external rotation injury. The direction of the spiral could have been predicted from the history of the injury. As will be elaborated upon later, this information is important in understanding the location of the soft tissue hinges and hence in planning a closed reduction of the fracture.

The Oblique Fracture

Clinical[2, 24, 25] and available experimental data[15] indicate that the oblique fracture is the result of a combination of compression, bending, and torsional loads, the two most important components probably being compression and torsion. The summation of these three forces is equivalent to a bending load about an oblique axis.

In his book *Ruminations of an Orthopaedic Surgeon*, Dr. George Perkins[25] emphasized that it is important to distinguish between the oblique and spiral fracture patterns. Not only are they produced by different loads but they also have different prognoses: the spiral fracture usually heals uneventfully, whereas the oblique fracture often ends in nonunion.

On superficial examination the oblique fracture has a radiological appearance quite like that of the spiral fracture (Fig. 1.6); however, on closer examination the difference becomes apparent. In the oblique fracture the ends are short and blunt and there is no vertical segment, whereas the spiral fracture has long, sharp, pointed ends and a vertical segment is always present. Dr. Perkins compared the radiological picture of the oblique fracture to a garden trowel, that of the spiral fracture to a fountain pen nib. He felt that the higher incidence of nonunion in the oblique fracture was due to the lack of stability of the fracture fragments. Stability is, of course, a function of both fracture configuration and the presence of soft tissue support, which can be used to maintain a reduction. As the next two sections will demonstrate, from a biomechanical viewpoint the oblique fracture represents a higher energy injury than does the simple spiral fracture and, hence, more soft tissue injury and consequently delays in healing could be anticipated.

MAGNITUDE OF LOAD

In dealing with long bone fractures, not only must the type of force be considered but also its magnitude. The energy which produces the fracture is dissipated in a number of ways. Some is lost in the process of deforming (straining) the bone, some through the actual breaking apart of the intermolecular bonds within the bone, i.e., producing the fracture, and the rest is dissipated in the soft tissues surrounding the bone. Obviously the greater the magnitude of the force, the higher its energy content and, hence, the more tissue destruction. Conversely, the more complex the fracture pattern (oblique, oblique transverse, butterfly, and

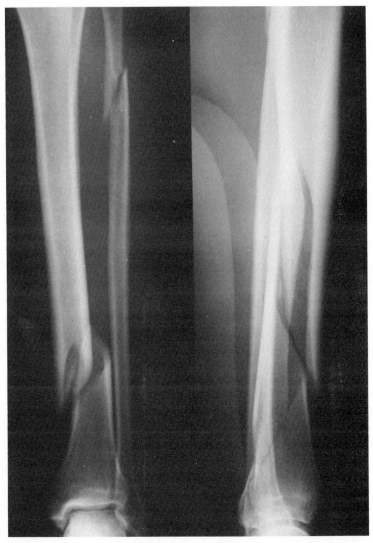

Figure 1.6. Comparison of oblique and spiral fractures of the tibia. The spiral fracture (*right*) has a tip like a fountain pen nib and a vertical segment, whereas the oblique fracture (*left*) is shaped like a garden trowel and has no identifiable vertical segment.[25] The distinction is important because oblique fractures are higher energy injuries and hence associated with a greater incidence of delayed union.

comminuted) the greater the energy needed to produce the fracture.[27] The fractures which result from these complex load configurations represent high energy injuries.

LOAD RATE

In recent years, students of fracture biomechanics have recognized the necessity of specifying the rate at which the force was applied (load rate) when discussing the results of biomaterials testing.[12, 18, 20, 22, 26, 28] This information is needed because bone and most other biological materials possess *viscoelastic* properties. A viscoelastic material is one whose mechanical properties vary according to how rapidly the forces are applied. For example, Sammarco et al.[28] showed experimentally that it requires approximately 43% more torsional energy to break diaphyseal bone in 50 msec than to break it in 150 msec. Not only is more energy required to produce the fracture but the energy imparted to the bone is not dissipated in an orderly manner.[16, 26, 28] Numerous secondary fracture lines are created by minor discontinuities, and the bone literally explodes. The radiological appearance is that of a comminuted fracture (Fig. 1.7).

MATERIAL PROPERTIES OF BONE

The orthopedist needs to understand the properties of bone as a material for the same reason that an architect needs to understand the characteristics of wood or concrete. A craftsman cannot appreciate the mechanical properties of the overall structure unless he has first acquired an intimate knowledge of the physical properties of the basic material. Because bone is the fundamental structural material of the skeleton, the orthopedist must understand both its strength and its inherent weakness if he is to deal logically with musculoskeletal injuries.

It is important to distinguish between the *material* and *structural* properties of bone. When talking about the material properties of bone, the physical properties of the bone itself are described, whereas when discussing the structural properties of bone, how size, shape, and configuration (i.e., structure) affect strength is described. Both of these concepts are important to the understanding of why a particular fracture pattern occurs.

A great deal of engineering effort has been expended in the study of the material properties of bone. The reader is encouraged to examine this important subject in the comprehensive review provided by Reilly and Burstein.[27] Although a detailed review is outside the scope of this book, this section will point out a few of the properties which distinguish bone from other structural materials. An engineer might define adult bone

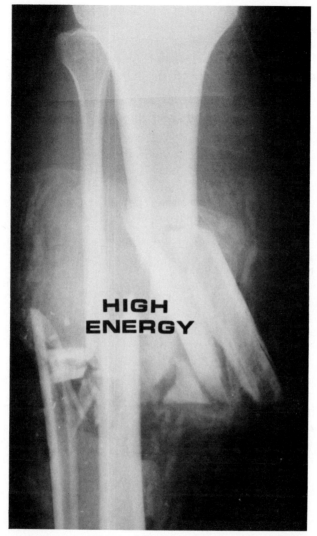

Figure 1.7. Comminuted tibia and fibular fracture as the result of a motorcycle accident. This high energy fracture with its associated soft tissue injuries eventually required amputation.

cortex as a nonhomogeneous, anisotropic, viscoelastic, brittle material which is weakest when loaded in tension. This definition, although somewhat overpowering, is seen to be quite straightforward when it is broken down into its components.

Nonhomogeneous

The mechanical properties of bone vary greatly depending on its type (tibia *versus* femur),[9] region (lateral *versus* medial cortex),[12] and nature (woven *versus* lamellar bone).[18] For this reason, values quoted for the mechanical properties of bone are meaningless unless the type of bone and the site from which it was removed are specified.

Anisotropic

A material is called "anisotropic" when it has different mechanical properties according to its orientation in the testing machine. For example, cortical bone is about twice as stiff when tension loads are applied parallel to the long axis of the bone as when such loads are applied at right angles.[27] Hence, when discussing the mechanical properties of bone it is important to know how the cortical sample is oriented in the testing machine.

Viscoelastic

As described in the section on "Load Rate," any material whose mechanical properties vary depending upon the rate at which the load is applied is called viscoelastic. Virtually all biological materials have this property and it exerts an important influence on fracture biomechanics.

Brittle

Because bone is brittle, it will, when deformed, break before other musculoskeletal materials. However, throughout the distance which it bends, it is elastic; i.e., it returns to its original shape when the load is released. Because it bends only slightly before breaking and because it is viscoelastic, bone is a poor absorber of shock loads. Its brittleness can be attributed to its mineral content,[10] and at high load rates it behaves like chalk.[3]

Weak in Tension

There is considerable experimental evidence to indicate that adult cortical bone is weaker under tension than under compressions loads,[3,11] and, as a consequence, most long bone fractures are the result of tension failure, whether this is produced by pure tension, bending, or torsional loads. How this characteristic influences fracture patterns is described under "Type of Load."

The properties noted above are important to the understanding of fracture biomechanics. One cannot accurately interpret experimental data on the mechanical properties of bone without appreciating its nonhomogeneous and anisotropic nature. Similarly, concepts such as viscoelasticity, brittleness, and tensile weakness are fundamental to understanding how long bones behave when they are subjected to various load configurations and strain rates. These are but a few of the physical properties that make bone a unique and fascinating material.

STRUCTURAL PROPERTIES OF BONE

It is meaningless to discuss fracture patterns and the material properties of bone without considering how these are influenced by shape. Some of the concepts that are important to an understanding of how structure affects the strength of a long bone include: 1) moment of inertia; 2) stress concentration; and 3) open and closed sections.

Moment of Inertia

Different shapes offer certain advantages in resisting bending or torsional loads. Obviously a wide hollow tube with thick walls can resist these forces more effectively than a thin solid rod (Table 1.2).

"Moment of inertia" is the engineering term which describes the degree to which the shape of a material influences its strength. There are two types of moment of inertia: the *area* moment of inertia describes rigidity to bending (bending resistance), and the *polar* moment of inertia describes rigidity to torsion (torsional resistance). Using mathematical techniques, the area and polar moments of inertia for an object of any shape can be calculated.

Table 1.2 shows the relative area moments of inertia of the same

Table 1.2.   Relative Resistance to Bending of Various Shapes

Shape		Relative Bending Resistance (Relative Area Moment of Inertia)^3
Solid rod		1
Flat beam (on end)		3.5
I beam (on end)		6
I beam (on side)		.6
Hollow cylinder		5.3

amount of material shaped as a rod, flat beam, I beam, and a hollow cylinder.[3] The I beam is the strongest shape (6 × solid rod), provided the bending load is applied to its strongest side, i.e., beam on end. If the load is applied with the I beam on its side, the strength is reduced by more than 90%. An engineer would say that the I beam is the strongest configuration for resisting unidirectional bending loads; hence, its popularity as a floor joist and its failure as a flag pole. As Table 1.2 illustrates, the more material located at a distance from the neutral axis, the greater its resistance to bending (area moment of inertia). Similarly, the more symmetrical an object with respect to its axis of rotation, and the more material that is situated at a distance from the neutral axis, the greater its resistance to torsional loads (polar moment of inertia).

Though the cylinder has a lower bending resistance than the I beam (Table 1.2), it has the advantage of having its mass arranged symmetrically about its neutral axis, i.e., a high polar moment of inertia. Consequently, the cylinder is the strongest structure for resisting combined bending and torsional loads. Perhaps for this reason, long bones have evolved as cylinders and not as I beams.

The concept of moment of inertia is also important because it explains why certain fractures are more common at specific sites. Figure 1.8, for example, shows a spiral fracture through the junction of the mid and distal one-third of the tibia resulting from a skiing injury. This is a common location for spiral tibial fractures. The drawings to the right of the line diagram show cross sections of the tibia at various levels. The cross section corresponding to the junction of the mid and distal third of the tibia (section *C*) shows that, although the cortex is thickest at this level, the outside diameter of the bone is narrowest here and its shape is somewhat triangular. Frankel and Burstein[15] calculated the moment of inertia at various sites along the tibia and found it to be lowest at the junction of the mid and distal one-third. They hypothesized that this low moment of inertia could account for the high incidence of fractures at this level.

Hence, the site at which a fracture occurs depends upon a number of factors, including the local thickness of the cortex, the material properties of the bone, and the overall geometry of the structure. The area and polar moments of inertia play an important role in fracture biomechanics because they are the physical parameters that describe the influence of geometry on long bone strength.

Stress Concentration

As just pointed out, the mechanical properties of bone are greatly influenced by its shape. For any structure, the mechanical properties will be least altered if one shape gradually blends into the next. Any sudden

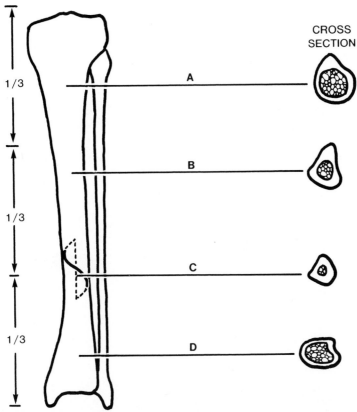

CROSS
SECTION

1/3

A

1/3

B

C

1/3

D

Figure 1.8. Spiral fracture junction mid and distal one-third tibia. The tendency for spiral fractures of the tibia to occur at the junction between the mid and distal one-third of the shaft can be explained by the low polar moment of inertia at this location.[15]

change in shape alters the distribution of stresses within the structure, giving rise to what engineers refer to as stress concentration (or stress risers). The stresses, which are a result of loading, can be thought of as analogous to the flow of water in a stream. Stress lines can be drawn to indicate the distribution of forces throughout the material, and this is analogous to the "flow" lines of water. In bone, the proximity of these stress lines to each other represents the stress concentration, whereas for a stream of water, the proximity of the flow lines represents the water velocity. A cortical screw hole or sudden change in contour is analogous to the presence of a large rock located in the middle of the stream. In order for the stress lines to pass around these discontinuities they must come closer together (i.e., increase the stress concentration), much as the flow lines must come closer in the stream (increasing the velocity of the water). If the local stress concentration exceeds the breaking point of the bone, a crack will form (Fig. 1.9) in the same way that waves or turbulence forms if the flow of the stream exceeds a certain velocity. The type of

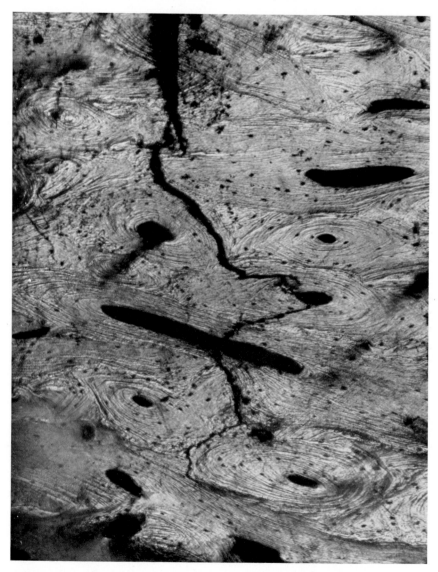

Figure 1.9.   Photo obtained through reflected light microscope illustrating propagation of crack through microconstituents of bone. Crack originated from stress riser (cortical defect) at top of picture.[26]

fracture pattern that develops will depend upon the other factors discussed earlier, i.e., type of force, magnitude of force, etc.

Bone remodels in response to forces to which it is subjected (Wolff's law: Form Follows Function[29]). It does this in such a way that its surface always presents a smooth contour with no abrupt changes in shape. A number of conditions can produce sudden changes in a bone's shape or material properties, resulting in stress concentration (Fig. 1.10). Common fractures that develop as a result of stress concentration include:

1. Pathological fracture through tumor;
2. Refracture near an area of callus;
3. Fracture at the end of a rigid internal fixation device; and
4. Fracture through a screw hole.

As internal fixation of bone fractures becomes more popular, we will probably see an increase in the number of refractures through screw holes following the removal of these devices. Experimentally, Laurence and associates[17] showed that diaphyseal drill holes produced up to a 40% loss of bending strength and a 12% loss of torsional strength. In similar experiments on dog long bone, Burstein et al.[7] showed a 55% reduction in energy absorption capacity under torsional loads. Bechtol and associates[3] demonstrated a 30% loss of bending strength as a result of drill holes on the tension side of the bone but *no* change in strength if the drill hole is placed on the compression side.

Burstein et al.[7] have studied the rate at which torsional strength returned following removal of screws from dog femurs. They found that the strength returned to normal within 8 weeks of removal of a screw, and that it returned at the same rate when the hole was left untouched, when it was redrilled to remove fibrous tissue, or when it was filled with a soft Silastic plug to prevent new bone formation. Their study indicates that bone rapidly remodels in an attempt to compensate for the effect of stress risers. This capacity is limited, however, and the bone requires considerable time to bring this about.

Because of stress concentration, the fractures through screw holes develop in response to much lower energies than are required to fracture intact bone; usually the crack is initiated by the hole.[7] The spiral and transverse fracture patterns that occur through screw holes are quite characteristic (Fig. 1.11). Note that when a spiral fracture develops because of torsional loading, the screw hole is usually at the midpoint of the spiral, directly opposite the vertical segment. A transverse fracture usually develops when the screw hole is under tension, and hence the hole is usually found opposite the concavity of the fracture.

Open and Closed Sections

Although the mechanical implications of open and closed sections relate to both moment of inertia and stress concentration, we have chosen

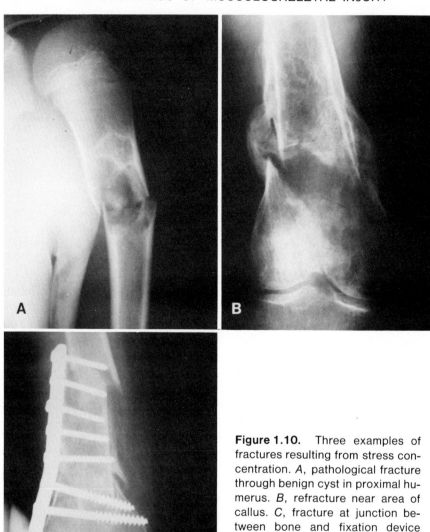

Figure 1.10. Three examples of fractures resulting from stress concentration. *A*, pathological fracture through benign cyst in proximal humerus. *B*, refracture near area of callus. *C*, fracture at junction between bone and fixation device (condylar plate).

to discuss this topic separately because it has a specific clinical significance.

The hollow cylinder is an excellent example of a *closed section* struc-

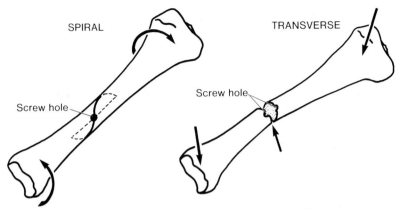

Figure 1.11. Fractures through screw holes.

ture. Because of its symmetry and the absence of any defects in its walls, all forces are dissipated evenly over its surface. This confers a great deal of structural rigidity to the cylinder. However, if a longitudinal section were removed from its wall, the cylinder would be converted to an *open section* and its strength greatly diminished.

For long bones, the mechanics of open and closed sections can be understood best by representing the internal resistance to torsional loads as closed loops of "stress" lines analogous to the flow of water in a conduit.[15] An intact diaphyseal bone can be thought of as a *closed section* because all of the stress lines set up in response to torsional loads flow in the same direction. On the other hand, if a vertical segment of cortex is removed (e.g., a bone graft donor site), the bone is converted to an *open section*. In this situation, the stress lines, in order to form a closed loop, have to return in the opposite direction along the inner cortex of the bone; the overall effect is to decrease the resistance to torsion. Experimentally, Frankel and Burstein[14] have shown that cutting a longitudinal slot in the diaphysis of long bone, i.e., converting it from a closed to open section, reduces the torsional strength by 80–90%.

Figure 1.12 shows a distal femoral fracture that occurred intraoperatively while treating an elderly woman's intertrochanteric hip fracture. The surgeon had elected to treat the hip fracture using the Enders technique (the underlying biomechanics of which are described in Ch. 2). This technique necessitates creating a *vertical slot* in the medial cortex of the distal femoral metaphysis, through which the Enders' nails are inserted. During a vigorous attempt to extract a maldirected nail, the femur fractured through the slot in the medial cortex. The distraught and apologetic orthopedic resident had failed to appreciate that the vertical slot in the medial metaphysis constituted an *open section* and hence was vulnerable to fracture.

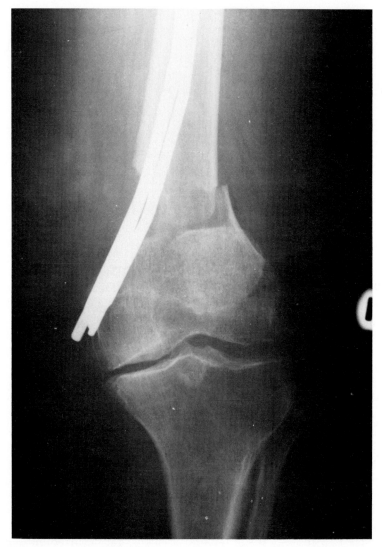

Figure 1.12. Fracture of distal femur that occurred intraoperatively through "open section" while extracting an Enders nail.

The surgeon should always be aware that when he removes a vertical segment of cortex from a long bone, he is converting the bone from a rigid closed section to a much weaker open section structure. Similarly it should be understood that the clover leaf intramedullary nail is an open section structure and hence should be inserted in a specific manner to reduce this effect. This latter aspect will be dealt with in greater detail in Chapter 3, "Biomechanics of Internal Fixation."

FRACTURE PATTERNS

This chapter has demonstrated that most long bone fractures develop in a predictable manner. All basic fracture patterns represent some combination of bending, torsion, or compression loads, as modified by the magnitude and rate of application of the load and the local characteristics of the bone—shape, presence of stress concentrations, etc. Hence, in assessing long bone fractures, the surgeon should always be aware of the five factors that determine the manner in which a long bone will fracture:

1. Type of load
2. Magnitude of load
3. Load rate
4. Material properties of bone
5. Structural properties of bone

Table 1.3 summarizes the biomechanics of long bone fractures. From the radiological fracture pattern one can determine the mechanism of

Table 1.3. Summary of Long Bone Fracture Biomechanics

Fracture Pattern	Appearance	Mechanism of Injury	Location Soft Tissue Hinge	Energy
Transverse		Bending	Concavity	Low
Spiral		Torsion	Vertical segment	Low
Oblique-transverse or butterfly		Compression + Bending	Concavity or side of butterfly	Mod
Oblique		Compression + Bending + Torsion	Concavity (often destroyed)	Mod
Comminuted		Variable	Destroyed	High
Metaphyseal compression		Compression	Variable	Variable

injury and the location of the soft tissue hinges and can estimate the amount of energy involved in producing the fractures. This figure gives an oversimplified view of fracture analysis because it is obvious that not all transverse or spiral fractures result from low energy forces and, conversely, not all complex fracture patterns result from high energy loads. However, biomechanically and clinically, certain fracture patterns are associated with high energy injury, and the observer should be aware of these patterns. The presence of a complex diaphyseal fracture pattern (oblique, oblique transverse, butterfly, comminuted) should alert the clinician to the possibility of soft tissue and neurovascular complications. If he trains himself to recognize these patterns and carries out a careful history and physical examination, he will anticipate and take appropriate measures to prevent these complications.

Knowing the position of the soft tissue hinges, the surgeon can manipulate the fracture to achieve stable reduction. The higher the energy involved, the greater the probability of disruption of the hinges, but, when present, their location can be predicted by the type of fracture pattern.[2] For transverse, oblique, and oblique transverse patterns the soft tissue hinges are located on the concavity of the fracture. For the butterfly and spiral patterns the hinges are found on the sides corresponding to the position of the butterfly fragment and vertical segment, respectively.

From the fracture pattern one can deduce the mechanism of injury, the amount of energy involved, and the location of the soft tissue hinges. The surgeon needs all this information before he can lay out a treatment protocol.

From the viewpoint of fracture biomechanics, not only is the type of load (compression, bending, torsion) important, but also its magnitude and rate of application. The two latter factors determine the amount of energy imparted to the bone and, hence, determine whether the force will result in one of the simple fracture patterns (i.e., transverse or spiral) or whether it will produce a severely comminuted fracture with extensive soft tissue destruction.

It is important to distinguish between the mechanical properties of bone as a *material* and as a *structure.*

As a *material* it is anisotrophic, viscoelastic, and brittle. The first two terms imply that its mechanical properties will vary markedly depending on the orientation of the bone and also upon how rapidly it is loaded. It is brittle because it bends very little before breaking.

When discussing bone as a *structure* one must also consider how shape and local surface irregularities affect strength. Shape has an important influence on the strength of bone. The quality that describes the bending resistance of bone is the area moment of inertia, and the one that describes its torsional resistance is the polar moment of inertia. An appreciation of these concepts has greatly added to our understanding of fracture biomechanicals because they explain why certain fractures develop at predictable locations and why certain forms of internal fixation are stronger than others.

The concept of stress concentration enables us to appreciate the effect of surface irregularities on bone strength. Because most of the long bone stress is distributed along its surface (away from the neutral axis), any sudden surface discontinuity can markedly increase the local stress within the bone. This effect is known as "stress concentration." If the local stresses exceed the yield point of the bone, a crack will form and propagate into a fracture. These fractures occur at much lower loads than would be necessary in the absence of a stress contraction.

Stress concentration may develop naturally, i.e., tumors or bone islands, or as a result of surgical intervention. As described earlier in the chapter, the process of internal fixation itself can produce stress concentration and secondary fractures. It has been shown that a single screw can reduce torsional and bending rigidity by almost 50% and that removal of a vertical segment of bone (resulting in the creation of an open section) can reduce bone strength more than 80%.

All of the factors mentioned above influence long bone fracture patterns, whether they result from combinations of high energy, bending or torsional loads acting on normal bone or lower energy loads acting through regions of local stress concentration. An understanding of long bone biomechanics allows the orthopedist to design a treatment protocol that is tailored to the "personality" of the individual fracture.

References

1. ALLEN WC, PIOTROWSKI G, BURSTEIN AH, et al: Biomechanical principles of intramedullary fixation. *Clin Orthop* 60:13–20, 1968.
2. ALMS M: Fracture mechanics. *J Bone Joint Surg* 43B:162–166, 1961.
3. BECHTOL CO: Engineering principles applied to orthopedic surgery. *Am Acad Orthop Surg Inst Course Lect* 9:257–264, 1952.
4. BECHTOL CO, FERGUSON AB, LAING PG: *Metals and Engineering in Bone and Joint Surgery*. Williams & Wilkins, Baltimore, 1959.
5. BECHTOL CO, MURPHY EF: The clinical application of engineering principles to the problems of fractures and fracture fixation. *Am Acad Orthop Surg Inst Course Lect* 9: 272–275, 1952.
6. BROOKS DB, BURSTEIN AH, FRANKEL VH: The biomechanics of torsional fractures. *J Bone Joint Surg* 52A:507–514, 1970.
7. BURSTEIN AH, CURREY J, FRANKEL VH, et al: Bone strength. The effect of screw holes. *J Bone Joint Surg* 54A:1143–1156, 1972.
8. BURSTEIN AH, REILLY DT, FRANKEL VH: Failure characteristics of bone and bone tissue. In *Perspectives in Biomedical Engineering*, edited by RM Kenedi. Macmillan, New York, 1973.
9. BURSTEIN AH, REILLY DT, MARTENS M: Aging of bone tissue: mechanical properties. *J Bone Joint Surg* 58A:82–86, 1976.

10. BURSTEIN AH, ZIKA JM, HEIPLE KG, et al: Contributions of collagen and mineral to the elastic-plastic properties of bone. *J Bone Joint Surg* 57A:956–961, 1975.
11. CURRY JD: Mechanical properties of bone. *Clin Orthp* 73:210–231, 1970.
12. EVANS FG, LEBROW M: Regional differences in some of the physical properties of the human femur. *J Appl Physiol* 3:563–572, 1951.
13. EVANS FG: Stress and strain in the long bones of the lower extremity. *Am Acad Orthop Surg Inst Course Lect* 9:264–271, 1952.
14. FRANKEL VH, BURSTEIN AH: Load capacity of tibular bone. In *Biomechanics and Related Bio-Engineering Topics*. Pergamon Press, New York, 1965.
15. FRANKEL VH, BURSTEIN AH: The biomechanics of refracture of bone. *Clin Orthop* 60:221–225, 1968.
16. HIRSCH C, CAVADIAS A, NACHEMSON A: An attempt to explain fracture type. *Acta Orthop Scand* 24:8–29, 1954.
17. LAURENCE M, FREEMAN MA, SWANSON SA: Engineering considerations in the internal fixation of fractures of the tibial shaft. *J Bone Joint Surg* 51B:754–768, 1969.
18. MATHER BS: Observations on the effects of static and impact loading on the human femur. *J Biomech* 1:331–335, 1968.
19. McELHANEY JH: Dynamic response of bone and muscle tissue. *J Appl Physiol* 21: 231–236, 1966.
20. McELHANEY J, BYERS EF: *Dynamic Response of Biological Materials*, 65-WA/ HUF-9. ASME Publications, 1965.
21. MURPHY EF: Engineering principles in fracture fixation. *Am Acad Orthorp Surg Inst Course Lect* 11:95–97, 1954.
22. PANJABI MM, WHITE AA, SOUTHWICK WO: Mechanical properties of bone as a function of rate of deformation. *J Bone Joint Surg* 55A:322–330, 1973.
23. PEDERSEN HE, SERRA JB: Injury to the collateral ligaments of the knee associated with femoral shaft fractures. *Clin Orthop* 60:119–121, 1968.
24. PERKINS G: *Fractures and Dislocations*. Athlone Press, London, 1958.
25. PERKINS G: *Ruminations of an Orthopaedic Surgeon*. Butterworths, London, 1970.
26. PIEKARSKI K: Fracture of bone. *J Appl Physiol* 41:1, 1970.
27. REILLY DT, BURSTEIN AH: The mechanical properties of cortical bone. *J Bone Joint Surg* 56A:1001–1021, 1974.
28. SAMMARCO GJ, BURSTEIN AH, DAVIS WL, et al: The biomechanics of torsional fractures: the effect of loading on ultimate properties. *J Biomech* 4:113–117, 1971.
29. WOLFF J: *Das Gaetz der Transformation. Transformation der Knocken*. Hirschwald, Berlin, 1892.

Questions—Chapter 1

1. Long bone fractures that result from torsional loads tend to follow a spiral course:
   a. 20° from the long axis
   b. 45° from the long axis
   c. 65° from the long axis
   d. 80° from the long axis

2. The effect of a diaphyseal screw hole on the bone in region of the hole is to:
   a. decrease its stiffness (elastic modulus)
   b. increase its stiffness (elastic modulus)
   c. decrease the stress concentration as compared with bone remote from the hole
   d. increase the stress concentration as compared with bone remote from the hole

3. Bone is said to be viscoelastic. This means that:
   a. its mechanical behavior is constant
   b. its mechanical behavior varies with the load rate
   c. the material is brittle but strong
   d. it contains a viscous (gelatinous) fluid

4. Adult cortical bone is strongest when subjected to:
   a. tension
   b. compression
   c. bending
   d. torsion

5. Increasing the strain rate from slow to fast will have what effect?
   a. decrease bone stiffness
   b. decrease energy absorption to failure
   c. increase energy absorption to failure
   d. no effect on the mechanical properties of bone

6. The capacity of a structure to have differing mechanical properties depending upon its rate of deformation, is described as:
   a. anisotropic
   b. viscoelastic
   c. brittle
   d. elastic

7.   Long bone fractures occur most frequently as the result of:
    a. fatigue
    b. compressive stress
    c. stiffness
    d. tensile stress

8.   The removal of a vertical slot cortical graft from a long bone (creating an "open section") reduces its torsional resistance by:
    a. 10%
    b. 25%
    c. 50%
    d. 80%

9.   The strongest shape to resist both torsion and bending is the:
    a. solid rod
    b. I beam
    c. flat beam
    d. cylinder

10.   Pure bending loads applied to a long bone would most probably produce the following fracture pattern:
    a. diaphyseal impaction
    b. transverse
    c. oblique transverse or butterfly
    d. spiral

11.   Combined bending and axial compression load applied to a long bone would most probably produce the following fracture pattern:
    a. diaphyseal impaction
    b. transverse
    c. oblique transverse or butterfly
    d. spiral

12.   When a long bone is subjected to a bending load, the neutral axis refers to:
    a. the region on the concavity of the bone (i.e., subjected to compression forces)
    b. the region on the convexity of the bone (i.e., subjected to tension forces)
    c. the region in the center of the bone (subjected to neither tension nor compression forces)
    d. the two end of the bone

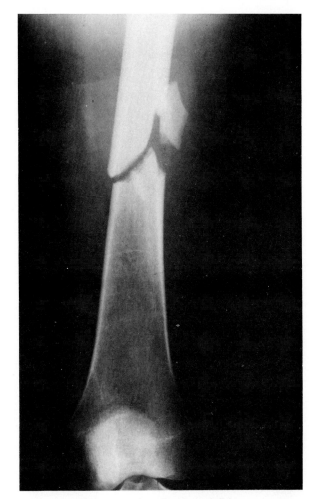

Figure 1.13. Fractured tibia.

13.   The femoral fracture shown in Figure 1.13 most probably resulted from the following load:
a. torsional
b. blow to medial aspect of thigh
c. blow to lateral aspect of thigh
d. axial compression (fall from height landing on heal)

14.   The area moment of inertia refers to:
a. how the shape of a material confers torsional rigidity
b. how the shape of a material confers bending rigidity

    c. how the rate of application of a load effects bending rigidity

    d. how the rate of application of a load effects torsional rigidity

15. The polar moment of inertia refers to:
    a. how the shape of a material confers torsional rigidity
    b. how the shape of a material confers bending rigidity
    c. how the rate of application of a load effects bending rigidity
    d. how the rate of application of a load effects torsional rigidity

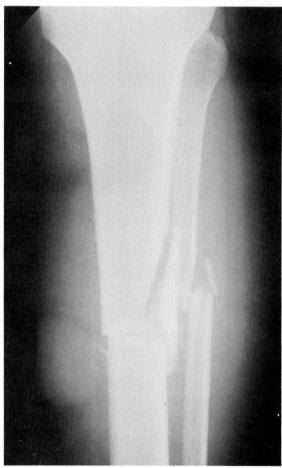

Figure 1.14. Fractured femur.

16. Torsional load applied to a long bone would be expected to produce:
    a. transverse fracture
    b. spiral oblique fracture
    c. comminuted fracture
    d. spiral fracture

17. Which history would be most compatible with the fracture configuration shown in the radiograph in Figure 1.14?
    a. fall from height, landing on heel of injured leg with knee and hip extended (i.e., axially applied load)
    b. external rotation injury resulting from tip of ski mogol
    c. blow to medial side of calf with foot firmly planted on ground
    d. blow to lateral side of calf with foot firmly planted on ground

1.3; see "Type of Load").

Bone"); 15) a (see "Structural Properties of Bone"); 16) d (see "Type of Load"); 17) d (Fig. 12) c (Fig. 1.2); 13) c (Fig. 1.3; see "Type of Load"); 14) b (see "Structural Properties of d (Frankel¹⁴); 9) d (see "Structural Properties of Bone"); 10) b (Fig. 1.2); 11) c (Fig. 1.3); 5) c (see "Load Rate"); 6) b (see "Load Rate"); 7) d (see "Material Properties of Bone"); 8) Answers—Chapter 1: 1) b (Fig. 1.8); 2) b (Burstein⁷); 3) b (see "Load Rate"); 4) b (Curry¹¹);

CHAPTER 2

Biomechanics of Joint Injuries

Ian J. Harrington

Injuries involving joints are common. Damage may occur to bony or soft tissue structures comprising the joint. The concept of a theoretical joint will assist the physician in analyzing injuries to the structures. Every joint, whether hip, knee, ankle, or finger, has definite anatomical components, namely, synovium and synovial fluid, articular cartilage, ligaments and joint capsule, and muscles spanning the joint.

Synovium and Synovial Fluid

The synovium provides synovial fluid for joint lubrication and for the norishment of cartilage. As in an engine, where all moving parts must be adequately lubricated to reduce friction, minimize heat production, and prevent wear between moving parts, so it is in human "bearings." The lubricating material in this case is synovial fluid produced by the joint lining. Traumatic damage to the synovium may produce hemarthrosis and a thickened, boggy, blood-stained synovium. Subsequently, adhesions may develop, restricting movement and producing joint stiffness.

Prolonged immobilization, by diminishing joint lubrication, also contributes to "fracture disease," namely, atrophy of muscle, cartilage, skeletal decalcification, atrophy of subcutaneous fat, capsular contraction, chronic circulatory disturbances, and stiffening of joints. When the synovium has been damaged, treatment (if possible) should aim at early restoration of movement so as to prevent adhesions and minimize joint stiffness.

Articular Cartilage

The articular cartilage has three major mechanical functions: it controls joint motion; it transmits force (load) from adjacent limb segments; and, by virtue of its specific configuration, it helps to maintain joint stability.

Control of Joint Motion

Control of joint motion is achieved through the shape of the joint's articular surface; for example, the hip and shoulder are ball-and-socket joints. Movement is not restricted to any particular plane; i.e., they are universal joints. By contrast, the knee and elbow are hinged joints and movement is restricted primarily to one plane. The shape, therefore, of the articular surfaces determines to a major degree the joint's movements, and these may be quite complex. At the knee, for example, during flexion extension, rolling and gliding occur synchronously and are combined with axial rotation. The center of rotation at the knee is constantly changing,[16] while the hip has a single point of rotation. The shoulder, like the hip, is a ball-and-socket joint, but the articular surfaces are less congruous. The greater the degree of freedom of movement thus achieved is at the expense of stability. It is much easier, for example, to dislocate the shoulder than the hip. It is apparent, then, that stability and movement are related.

Joint Stability

Joint stability depends to some degree on the shape of its bearing surfaces. In most joints, two surfaces are mated one against the other: one surface is usually convex (male) and the other concave (female). The bearing surfaces of a joint tend to be congruous; i.e. the male and female parts of the joint are mated together. There are varying degrees of congruity. The hip, for example, has highly congruous surfaces where the concave acetabular component is closely matched to the convex femoral head. The femoral head is deeply seated in the acetabulum so that the joint's specific shape renders it inherently stable. The articular surfaces of the knee, by contrast, are not closely mated: the femoral condyles are convex and articulate, with relatively flat tibial plateaus. Thus, the knee is inherently unstable. Such stability as it has is provided by the strong ligaments and muscles which connect its components.

Load Transmission (Bearing Loads)

Generally, when bearing surfaces are congruous, stress distribution (force per unit of area) tends to be more uniform and of less magnitude, because the area of contact between congruent joint surfaces is greater than for surfaces that are poorly mated. It should be emphasized that the area of joint contact under load is most important and anything which disturbs or alters the surface contact area will increase stress concentration in the joint. As is well known, joints which have incongruous articular surfaces either from disease or trauma are predisposed to degenerative change, particularly major weight-bearing joints, such as the hip, knee, and ankle. It is a fundamental orthopedic principle that all intra-articular fractures, particularly those that involve major weight-bearing joints, must be reduced and stabilized to restore normal joint contour (Fig. 2.1 A and B). Displaced intra-articular fractures which are not anatomically

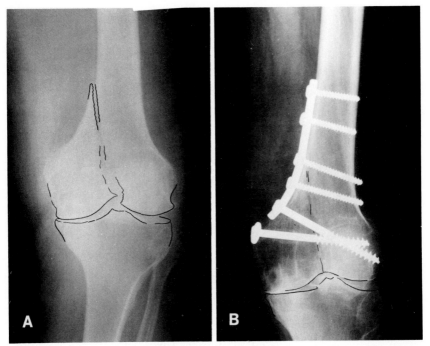

Figure 2.1. *A* and *B*, intra-articular fractures of major weight-bearing joints require restoration of the articular surfaces to restore normal joint contour. This is necessary in order to avoid stress risers in the joint.

reduced eventually produce degenerative changes because of the increased intra-articular stress concentrations.

Ligaments and Joint Capsule

Ligaments and joint capsular structures play a major role in stabilizing joints. Joints with relatively incongruous articular surfaces usually have strong collateral ligaments to resist force transmission across the joint. In the knee, for example, strong collateral ligaments resist abduction—adduction loads, and cruciate ligaments resist anteroposterior forces[6] (Fig. 2.2). As well as stabilizing a joint, ligaments transmit load from one limb segment to another[24, 42] (see *Ligaments* under "Knee Joint").

Muscles

The most obvious role of muscles is to move limb segments, but other important functions are to stabilize the joint and absorb energy during load transmission. During gait, for example, the muscles transmit load smoothly from one limb segment to another, thereby eliminating sharp

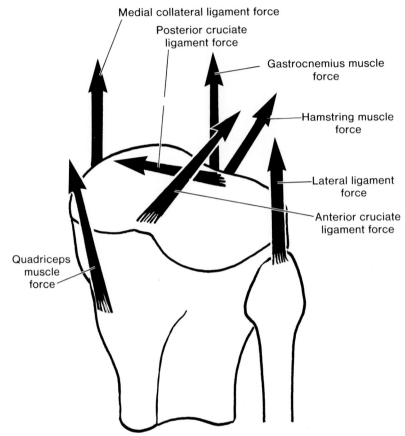

Medial collateral ligament force

Posterior cruciate ligament force

Gastrocnemius muscle force

Hamstring muscle force

Lateral ligament force

Anterior cruciate ligament force

Quadriceps muscle force

Figure 2.2.   Bending moments and forces applied to a joint are transmitted from limb segment to segment by muscle and ligaments spanning the joint.

force peaks.[48] A major part of the difficulty in simulating fracture patterns relates to the difficulty of reproducing muscle action experimentally.

SIMPLE BIOMECHANICS

To understand the biomechanics of joint injuries, the reader must be familiar with certain simple mechanical concepts,[59] namely, the lever, bending or turning moments, and stress and stress concentration. *The lever* has many applications in orthopedic surgery, for example, to gain mechanical advantage. The greater the distance between the fulcrum and the point of application of the force, as in a first class lever, the easier it is to lift a weight. Levers are classified as first, second, and third class, according to the point of application of the applied force, the position of the fulcrum, and the object to be moved.

In the *first class* lever, the fulcrum is situated between the applied load and the resisting weight (W) or object. In Figure 2.3, the applied force (F) multiplied by its lever arm, i.e., the distance from the force to the fulcrum, must equal the weight of the object, multiplied by its lever arm, the distance from the fulcrum to the weight. The ratio of the lever arms determines the mechanical advantage. The greater the lever arm (*a*), the less force required to lift the weight.

In the *second class* lever (Fig. 2.4), the weight is located between the applied force and the fulcrum. The ankle joint frequently works as a second class lever. When a person stands on tiptoes, the fulcrum is located where the ball of the foot touches the ground; the force applied through the gastrocnemii acts at the ankle, lifting body weight (Fig. 2.4).

With the *third class* lever (Fig. 2.5), the applied force is always located between the fulcrum and supported weight. In the upper extremity, the biceps insertion is located between the elbow joint and the hand. When lifting a weight, the biceps contracts with the elbow joint as the fulcrum. Here, the load arm is longer than the effort arm so that the mechanical advantage is small and hence is not as efficient as the first and second class levers.

The first class lever is a common system in human joints. For example, at the hip the body's weight is balanced over the joint by the abductor muscles acting through the greater trochanter[33] (Fig. 2.6). Similarly, during ambulation, body weight acts medial to the knee so that the center of rotation (the fulcrum) is centered over the medial condyle.[24, 42] Here equilibrium is maintained by a force acting in the lateral ligament complex (lateral ligament, tensor fascia, and biceps femoris) (Fig. 2.7). As will be explained during the analysis of specific joint injuries, the lever system has many applications to gait mechanics.

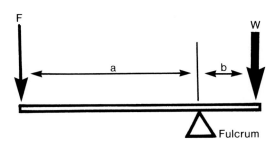

Figure 2.3. A simple first class lever. The applied force multiplied by its lever arm equals the weight of the object multiplied by its lever arm, the distance from the fulcrum to the weight. The mechanical advantage is related to the ratio of the lever arms *a* and *b*.

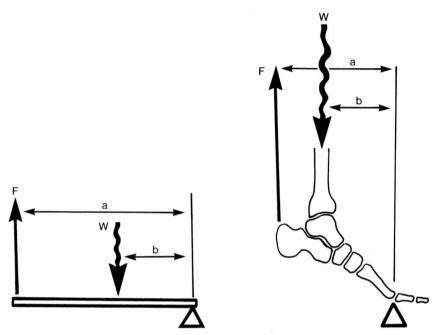

Figure 2.4. A second class lever system at the ankle. Body weight is located between the applied force and the fulcrum. The fulcrum is located where the ball of the foot touches the ground.

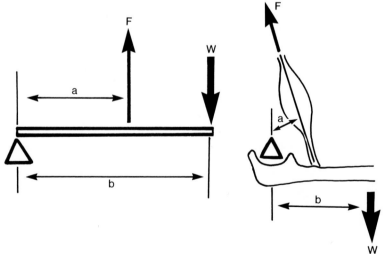

Figure 2.5. With a third class lever, the applied force is located between the fulcrum and supported weight. The mechanical advantage is small and the system is not as efficient as a first or second class lever system.

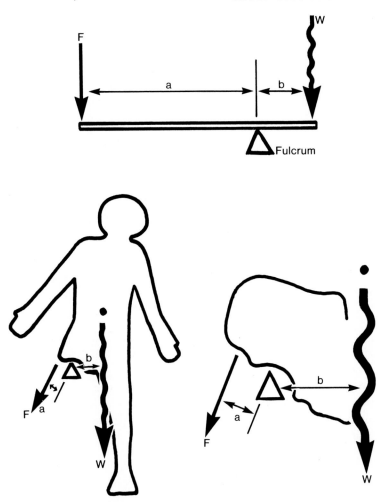

Figure 2.6.   The hip acts as a first class lever. Body weight is balanced over the hip joint (fulcrum) by abductor muscle pull. The mechanical advantage is related to the ratio of the lever arms *a* and *b*.

The Bending Moment (Torque)

When a force acts on an object, it has two effects: it will tend to move the object in the direction of its application (*translation*) and it will cause the object to turn or rotate (*turning* or bending moment). In the first class lever system at the hip, for example, body weight acting through the center of gravity tends to rotate the trunk towards the midline. This turning effect about the hip is due to body weight, and for equilibrium it

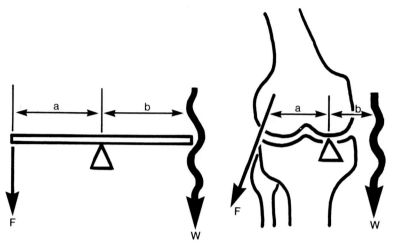

Figure 2.7. During normal gait the knee functions as a first class lever. Body weight is balanced by tensile force in the lateral tension band (lateral collateral ligament and tensor fascialata). The fulcrum is located on the medial joint compartment, and maximum joint force occurs here.

must be balanced by an equal and opposite turning effect by the abductor muscles pulling downwards on the pelvis. In each case the bending moment is the product of force multiplied by the perpendicular distance from the force to the center of rotation. In this example, the center of rotation is the hip joint. In every case, the turning effect or moment of the force is calculated using the perpendicular distance from the point of rotation to the applied force.

Stress and Stress Concentration

Stress is force per unit area expressed as pounds per square inch, kilograms per square centimeter, or any convenient measuring system. Stresses may be compression, tension, or shear, depending on whether the object is compressed, pulled apart, or sheared (Fig. 2.8). For a given force, the area over which it is applied determines the magnitude of stress or stress concentration.[53] The stress concentration on a linoleum floor from a stiletto heel, for example, is higher than for the same individual wearing a regular shoe with a wide based heel.

Obviously, stress concentration is a function of shape. Joints that are congruous have a relatively large area of bearing contact, so that stress concentration tends to be low. This factor also depends to some degree on the type of bearing material in contact under load; material such as cartilage, which is plastic and capable of deformation, decreases stress concentration by increasing the bearing surface area. (see Ch. 4).

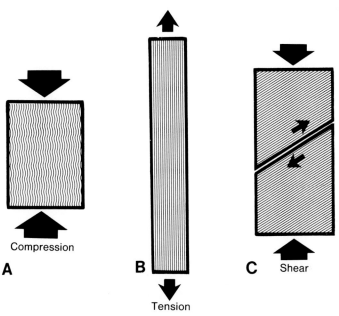

Figure 2.8. Stress and strain concentration. Stresses may be due to compression (*A*), tension (*B*), or shear (*C*) forces. The area over which a force is applied determines the magnitude of the stress. Tensile and compression stresses occur on a plane at right angles to the applied force. Shear stresses occur parallel to the plane considered. Maximum shear stresses occur on a plane inclined at 45° to the line of action of the major compressive or tensile force. Strain is the resulting deformation that occurs in a material subjected to stress.

Bending moments and stress are related. When a force is applied to the femoral head, for example, it tends to bend the femur so that the inner cortex is under compression and the lateral cortex is under tension. In 1917, Koch[37] showed that under this type of loading the subtrochanteric region of the femur undergoes maximum compression and tensile stress (Fig. 2.9).

The analysis of joint injuries requires an understanding of the lever system, bending moments, and stress concentration.

BIOMECHANICS OF JOINT INJURIES

Hip

Paul[47, 49, 50] and Rydell[54] have shown that during ambulation force across the hip joint may be three to five times the body weight and it increases considerably during activities more vigorous than walking. The forces transmitted during trauma have never been measured, but presum-

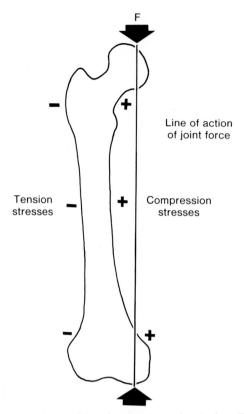

Figure 2.9. Compression and tension stresses due to bending of the femur. Normal loading of the femur due to bearing forces at the knee and hip as shown in this diagram results in bending of the femur, so that the bone fibers are compressed on the medial side and stretched laterally. Compression stresses are, therefore, maximal along the medial femoral cortex and tensile stresses are maximal in the lateral femoral cortex. The subtrochanteric region of the femur is subjected to the greatest compression and tensile stresses. *F*, joint force.

ably they are far greater than those generated during ambulation, particularly when force is applied suddenly (impact loading). The most common hip joint injury, fracture, is of three types: subcapital, intertrochanteric, and subtrochanteric.

These fractures usually occur during a fall and presumably are due to a combination of axial compression, torsion, shear, and bending loads. However, it is not clear, clinically or experimentally, why these specific fractures occur biomechanically.[15]

Subcapital Fractures

As Figure 2.10 demonstrates, the resultant hip joint force acting on the femoral head has two major components relative to the femoral neck: a *shear* force and *compression*. The bending moment due to the applied force is small because the distance from the subcapital region to the line of action of the hip joint force is short. These forces have three effects at the fracture surface.[21-23] Compression acts to impact the femoral head on the neck, thus increasing stability at the fracture line; shear acts to

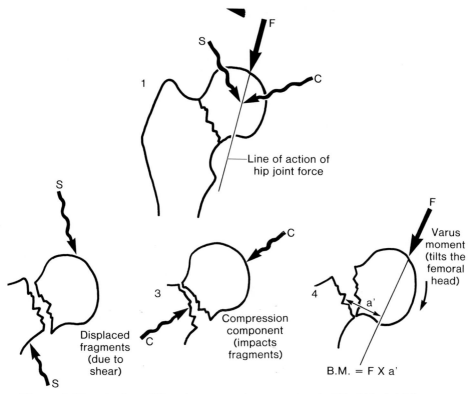

Figure 2.10. *1*, shear (*S*) and compression components (*C*) of hip joint force (*F*). Hip joint force has two major components. *2*, a shear component acts approximately parallel to the subcapital fracture line. Its effect is to displace the femoral head downwards relative to the femoral shaft. *3*, the other component, a compression force, acts perpendicular to the fracture line. Its effect is to compress the femoral lead against the neck of the femur. *4*, the hip joint force also has a moment effect, but this is small, since the lever arm (*a'*) is not great. Nevertheless, the moment effect is to tilt the head into a varus position. *B.M.*, bending moment.

displace the head relative to the neck in a direction parallel to the fracture surface; and the torque effect of joint force tilts the femoral head into varus.

Pauwels[52] classified subcapital fractures into three types, depending on the angle between the fracture line and the horizontal. In the anteroposterior radiograph, the more nearly vertical the fracture line, the greater its instability due to the effect of shear (type III fracture). The stable type I fracture has a more nearly horizontal fracture line; here, shear effect is negligible and compression predominates, impacting the head and neck fragments. The bending effect of the resultant joint force is small and not as important as the shearing factor (Fig. 2.11); it is approximately the same for both type I and type III fractures.The type II fracture is intermediate between types I and III.

Garden[18, 19] has classified subcapital fractures into four types, ranging from the essentially undisplaced impacted type I to the completely displaced type IV fracture. Garden's classification correlates the degree of displacement of the fracture before operation with the outcome after reduction and internal fixation. This classification, which is based on biological rather than mechanical criteria, has become very popular. Garden's excellent studies are highly recommended to any surgeon who deals with hip fractures.

Intertrochanteric Fractures

The mechanical factors noted above also apply to intertochanteric fractures. This type of fracture has been classified in several ways, but it

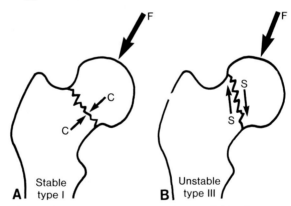

Figure 2.11. Pauwel's classification of subcapital hip fractures. *A*, type I fractures are stable because the fracture line tends to be horizontal so that the effect of joint force is to compress the femoral head against the neck of the femur. *B*, type III fractures are unstable because the fracture line tends to be vertical. This fracture displaces easily owing to shearing across the fracture surface.

is most practical to divide these fractures into stable and unstable injuries. Stable fractures are those in which the two major fragments are approximated in a position close to the anatomical norm. Unstable fractures are comminuted and it is difficult to achieve continuity between major fragments. The least stable ("four-part") fracture is made up of the head and neck, lesser and greater trochanters, and shaft (Fig. 2.12).[9, 10, 29] The force acting on the femoral head during weight bearing bends the shaft so that the medial cortex is compressed and the lateral cortex is under tension. During ambulation, the force acting on the femoral head may be three or four times the body weight. It should be noted further that the medial and lateral cortex stresses will be proportional to the length of the lever arm (Fig. 2.13). The moment at the fracture site for intertrochanteric fractures, therefore, is much greater than for subcapital fractures. At the intertrochanteric level, the resultant joint force acting on the femoral head has two major effects (Fig. 2.14), axial compression, and bending.

Shear is not a major consideration, but the axial rotation (torsion) imposed on the femoral shaft during internal and external rotation of the limb is a significant factor. These mechanical factors should be considered in the treatment of intertrochanteric fractures, particularly unstable ones.

Subtrochanteric Fractures

Subtrochanteric fractures are frequently associated with communication and loss of the medial cortical buttress. Mechanically, these are similar to intertrochanteric fractures except that the fracture contact area is much reduced, thus increasing the tendency to bending and rotational instability (Fig. 2.15). The most critical mechanical factor to

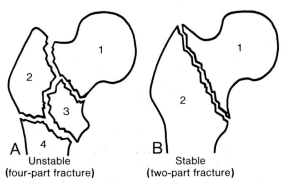

A Unstable
(four-part fracture)

B Stable
(two-part fracture)

Figure 2.12. Intertrochanteric fractures. *A*, unstable intertrochanteric fractures tend to be comminuted. The so called four-part fracture (head and neck, greater and lesser trochanter, and shaft segments) is the most common example of an unstable intertrochanteric fracture. *B*, two-part fractures are stable owing to continuity between the two major fracture segments.

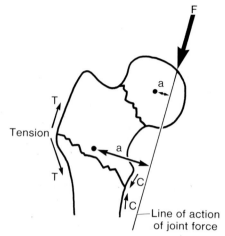

Figure 2.13.   The effect of hip joint force (*F*) on bending at subcapital and trochanteric levels. The greatest bending effect occurs at the intertrochanteric level owing to the long lever arm (*a*). Because of the bending effect, compression (*C*) stresses occur in the medial cortex and tensile stresses laterally. The bending effect of joint force is not as great at the subcapital level owing to the smaller bending moment lever arm (*a*). *T*, tension.

be accounted for in treatment is comminution, particularly medially, which destroys the normal medial buttress. The buttress should be reconstituted in order to prevent implant failure and avoid delayed union or nonunion of the fracture.

Koch[37] has shown that compression stresses are maximal in the subtrochanteric and proximal medial femoral shaft, the area where comminution occurs. If the medial cortices are not approximated at the time of surgical fixation, high bending stresses will be transmitted to the fixation device, increasing the risk of mechanical failure.

BIOMECHANICAL PRINCIPLES OF TREATMENT OF HIP FRACTURES

Subcapital Fracture

As previously described, subcapital fractures range from stable impacted to completely displaced. As in all fractures, the basic principle of treatment is to obtain and maintain a reduction, usually by means of internal fixation. The fixation device should achieve three things. It should resist shear stresses acting parallel to the fracture line; it should resist bending; and it should allow for axial compression.

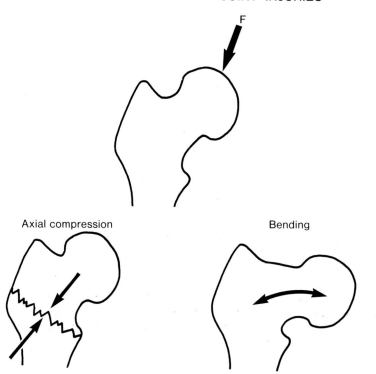

F

Axial compression   Bending

Figure 2.14.   The main effect of joint force at the trochanteric level. The resultant hip joint force (*F*) has two major effects at this level—axial compression and bending.

A variety of devices have been used, including threaded pins, solid and, more recently, sliding nails, but the specific device may not be as important as the mechanical principle behind its insertion. In low angle nail fixation (Fig. 2.16), the nail is placed to lie along the line of action of the resultant joint force.[20] Therefore, the bending moment on the nail is minimal, and the fracture surfaces rather than the nail bear the axial compression, so that this position reduces direct stress on the implant. As the fracture consolidates under compression loading, the nail often "backs" out through the lateral femoral cortex—a condition known as controlled collapse. Frankel[14] has shown experimentally that fixation can be enhanced by combining low angle fixation with an oblique nail or screw. Insertion of the screw corresponds to the tensile trabecular pattern of the femoral head and neck, whereas the low angle nail corresponds to the compression trabeculae (Fig. 2.17). Cross screw fixation (triangula-

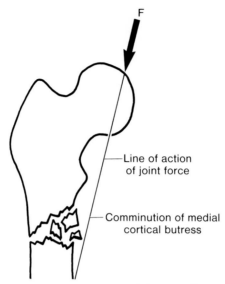

Figure 2.15. Subtrochanteric fractures of the hip. These fractures are frequently associated with communication and loss of the medial cortical buttress. The bony contact area at this level is small. Both factors contribute to bending and rotational instability.

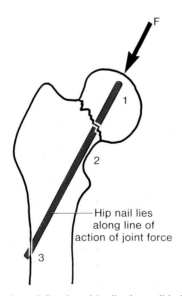

Figure 2.16. Low angle nail fixation. Ideally the nail is inserted along the line of action of the hip joint force (*F*). Bending stress on the implant therefore is minimal. The nail is supported at the femoral head (*1*), calcar (*2*) and lateral femoral cortex (*3*).

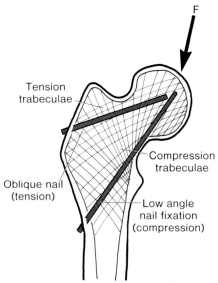

Figure 2.17. Two-nail (combination) fixation of hip fractures. Hip fracture fixation, particularly for the subcapital fracture, is enhanced with two-nail fixation. The low angle nail corresponds to compression trabeculae of the head-neck-trochanteric region, whereas the second nail corresponds to the tensile trabecular pattern. *F*, resultant hip joint force.

tion), based on the trabecular pattern of the proximal femur, has been used successfully by Smyth et al.[62] Horizontal nailing alone is unsatisfactory; when the nail lies in the "false axis" of the neck the bending moment is increased and encourages displacement of the head. Some workers have suggested that in the lateral plane the nail should be inserted into the posterior portion of the femoral head[22] because the nail tends to displace anteriorly during ambulation. Nailing of subcapital fractures that is based on biomechanical principles will have the following characteristics.

1. Low angle insertion so that the line of the nail corresponds closely to the line of action of the hip joint force. Under these conditions, the nail has three points of support: in the head; against the firm calcar it is buttressed midially; and it is embedded in the firm lateral cortex of the shaft.

2. Controlled collapse. Under axial load the nail should be extruded rather than penetrating into the hip joint.

3. Posterior inferior insertion of the nail.

Completely Displaced Subcapital Fracture

The completely displaced (garden Type IV) subcapital fracture is frequently complicated by avascular necrosis of the femoral head following closed reduction and pin fixation. For this reason, many surgeons prefer to remove the femoral head and insert an endoprosthesis of the Moore or Thompson variety. However, others advocate closed reduction and internal fixation of these fractures.

Figure 2.18*A* offers a simplified biomechanical analysis of the Moore type implant. The stem of the prosthesis is inserted into the intramedullary canal, thus securing it to the femoral neck and shaft. The prosthesis is so designed that its shoulder or collar abuts against the femoral neck. During weight bearing, the head of the prosthesis is loaded by the resultant joint force, and its line of action will be approximately the same as in the normal hip. Again, the prosthesis will be exposed to an axial compression and shear force component. The resultant hip force also causes a bending moment which tends to rotate the prosthesis into a varus position. This is a first class lever system in which the point of

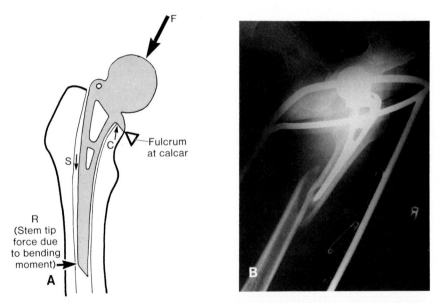

Figure 2.18. *A*, simplified biomechanics of an Austin-Moore prosthesis. During weightbearing, the head of the prosthesis is loaded so that the effect of the resultant joint force (*F*) is to tilt the prosthesis into a varus position. The calcar acts as a fulcrum and resistance to bending occurs because the stem tip abuts against the lateral femoral cortex. This is a first class lever system. The hip joint force also has the effect of causing compression (*C*) loading at the calcar and shear (*S*) along the interface between the metal stem and femoral shaft cortex. *B*, fracture of the femur after unipolar arthroplasty. This fracture pattern may be caused by high stress concentration on bone occurring in the region of the prosthetic stem tip.

contact between the shoulder of the prosthesis and the bony calcar acts as the fulcrum. As the prosthesis tilts into varus, the stem tip abuts against the lateral femoral cortex. As would be anticipated, stress concentrations on the bone around the prosthesis are high at the points of contact, namely, the region of the calcar and stem tip. Fractures of the femur following unipolar arthroplasty may be due to this loading mechanism, i.e., high stress concentrations at the tip of the prosthetic stem (Fig. 2.18B).

The compression component is transmitted by the collar of the prosthesis. If the fit between the prosthetic stem and medullary canal of the femur is snug, some of the compression will be transmitted via this mechanism. When the prosthesis is cemented into bone, axial loading will be transmitted partly to the collar and partly as "interface shear" between cement and bone.

Intertrochanteric Fractures

Biomechanically, intertrochanteric fractures may be stable or unstable, depending on the fracture pattern. Usually these fractures are treated by open reduction and fixation, using a nail plate combination. An understanding of the underlying mechanics is essential for the correct management of these injuries.

The first successful implant for hip fractures was the triflanged nail of Smith-Petersen.[61] Although others (e.g., Senn[60] in 1883) had used internal metallic fixation earlier, Smith-Petersen was the first to succeed, primarily because his nail was made of noncorrosive stainless steel. Initially he used the nail alone to treat fractures, but this did not prevent the head and neck fragments from drifting into varus or prevent rotation of the femoral shaft. Eventually a side plate was added, and since then a great variety of nail plate combinations have been used. The most recent is the sliding nail (screw) plate combination.

A successful nail plate must incorporate the following mechanical factors:

Bending—varus-valgus angulation (bending) of the head, must be prevented.

Rotation of the femoral shaft relative to the head and neck, must be controlled also.

Axial compression—forces must be transmitted from the head and neck to the shaft (impaction through controlled collapse). Ideally, most of the load should be taken up by the bone rather than the implant.

Shear stress acts parallel to the fracture surfaces. With impaction, shear is absorbed by the fracture surfaces rather than the implant, but the implant must be strong enough to resist the shear.

Traditionally, treatment of intertrochanteric hip fractures, whether stable or unstable, has aimed at anatomical restoration during reduction followed by fixation using a nail plate combination. This method is still in wide use,[26-28] but other methods have been introduced, chiefly because of complications related to unstable fractures. As Dimon and Hughston[9, 10, 29] point out, unstable intertrochanteric fractures do not have the support that comes from continuity of the bony cortex on the apposing surfaces of the proximal and distal fragments, either because of comminution of the medial aspect of the neck (calcar) or because of a posterior defect due to a separate trochanteric fragment. Often a fracture presents a combination of the two. If these fractures are not recognized as unstable[12] and if appropriate measures are not taken to restore stability, treatment may fail from the following causes: penetration of the nail into the hip; fracture of the nail; cutting out of the nail; cutting out of the plate.

In each situation, the mechanical cause of failure is the same, i.e., lack of a medial or posterior buttress producing excessive bending stress at the fracture plane (Fig. 2.19). Often this fracture configration is responsible for the unstable "four-part" intertrochanteric fracture. The restoration of biomechanical integrity requires reconstitution of the medial and posterior buttress by opposing the two major fragments, i.e., the head and neck segment to the femoral shaft. Hughston[30] recommends medial displacement of the femoral shaft combined with resection of the proximal bone spike to achieve stability (Fig. 2.20).

Since the hip joint force bends the head-neck segment into a varus position, it is desirable to reduce the hip in valgus. Dimon and Hughston[9, 10] assert that medial displacement fixation reduces the tendency of

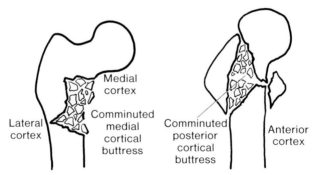

Figure 2.19.   Fracture instability of the hip due to disruption of the medial and posterior cortical buttresses. *A*, anteroposterior and *B*, lateral view. This fracture configuration is frequently responsible for the unstable four-part intertrochanteric fracture.

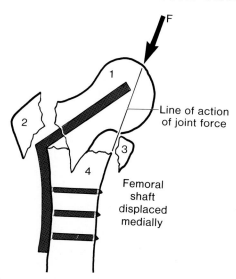

Figure 2.20. Medial displacement of unstable intertrochanteric fractures. The greater and lesser trochanters are ignored. The femoral shaft is displaced medially (*4*) so that the head-neck segment (*1*) is impaled in the medullary canal of the proximal femur. Mechanically this decreases the bending moment lever arm and impacts the two major fragments. *F*, joint force.

unstable fractures to develop a varus deformity after fixation. Biomechanically, this approach to fracture stability has logic on its side.

It should be emphasized that stress on the fixation appliance is greater in intertrochanteric fractures than in subcapital injuries chiefly because of the greater bending effect of hip joint force on the trochanteric region. With comminuted fractures, of course, inherent stability of bone is lost and the stress on the implant due to bending is correspondingly high. When the fracture is well reduced and impacted, most of the load will be transmitted by the bone rather than the nail, an important consideration.

Hip Fixation Devices

Rigid Nail Plate System

The main disadvantage of this type of nail plate is that it does not allow for controlled collapse of the fracture. If the fracture is not adequately reduced, i.e., the major fracture surfaces are not in contact and/or bone resorbs at the fracture line, the nail may penetrate the head, entering the hip joint. The nail may also bend or break due to high bending stresses, which are usually maximal at the nail plate junction. Also, varus angulation of the head and neck may develop with cutting out of the nail.

Sliding Nails

The sliding nail was devised in an attempt to overcome the disadvantages of the rigid nail plate system. Its main advantage is that it permits controlled collapse of the fracture and thus improves stability (Fig. 2.21). Compression can also be applied across the fracture site when a compression device like the Richard's screw plate combination is used at the time of surgery. The screw grips the head-neck fragment[25] so that compression can be applied, and as the screw slides within the barrel of the fixed angled plate, it allows controlled collapse of the fracture with weight bearing.

Intramedullary Nails

Intramedullary fixation of intertrochanteric fractures is achieved by flexible rods introduced through the medial femoral cortex in the region of the knee, upwards into the head and neck, across the fracture area.[8, 11, 38] The main biomechanical advantage is that there is less bending of the implant because this maneuver reduces the length of the bending moment lever arm (Fig. 2.22).

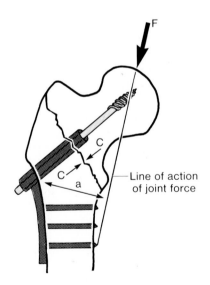

Figure 2.21. The mechanics of the sliding nail. The head and neck segment is firmly secured by the nail. Controlled collapse of the fracture is possible owing to sliding of the screw in the barrel of the plate device. This promotes compression (*C*), forces across the fracture surface. The bending moment on device (*F* × *a*) becomes smaller with controlled collapse, further increasing fracture stability.

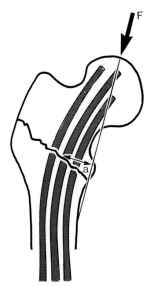

Figure 2.22. The mechanics of intramedullary nail fixation of fractures about the hip. The applied load is theoretically distributed over the full length of the femur, and stresses on the implants due to bending are reduced (*B.M. F × a*) because of the small bending moment lever arm.

Because nail plate devices are attached to the lateral cortex of the femur, the load is borne at the end of a long lever arm so that a large bending moment results. With flexible pins, the lever arm is shorter and the bending stresses less because the pins are closer to the line of action of the hip joint force. Theoretically, during weight bearing, load is distributed throughout the full length of the pins and evenly over the thigh as compared to local force concentration at the hip with a pin and plate. If properly inserted, the pins are positioned in a fan-shaped distribution in the femoral head, providing stability against rotation. This method of fracture fixation is new and requires further clinical evaluation to determine its final place in fracture treatment.

Subtrochanteric Fractures

Normal weight bearing produces high compression stresses in the subtrochanteric region because of the large bending moments in this region.[37, 51] Thus the management of a fracture in this area presents special problems.[13] If the fracture is stable with abutment of bone fragments, there is firm contact across the fracture plane. If a pin and plate device is applied to maintain reduction, compression stresses occur on the medial side at the area of bone contact and the plate will act as a tension band. If the fracture is comminuted or poorly reduced, the medial buttress may be absent. When this happens, the plate must resist most of the bending load and fatigue failure of the plate frequently develops (Fig. 2.23). A major disadvantage of a pin plate device for this fracture is that it does not allow the main fracture fragments to engage in "controlled collapse."

Because of the limitations of pin plate fixation for subtrochanteric fractures, considerable work has been done to develop intramedullary implants. Although the same mechanical principles apply to intramedullary fixation, bending stresses are usually lower because the distance from the femoral head to the central part of the rod is shorter. Also, during weight bearing, the fracture fragments can settle around the nail, making possible controlled collapse, a feature that is particularly important when the medial buttress has been lost. The risk of appliance failure is less because bending stresses developed in the implant are lower than those developed in a plate. Also it appears that the intramedullary nail carries less load than the plate, so that there is less disuse osteoporosis. Chapter 3 provides a further discussion of the phenomenon of stress protection. However, the intramedullary rod cannot prevent varus or valgus angulation of the head-neck-trochanteric region when the proximal

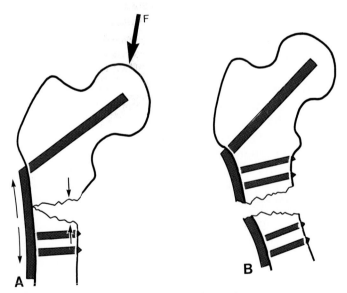

Figure 2.23.   Fixation device failure with subtrochanteric fractures. When the medial cortical buttress is absent because of comminution, the plate is subjected to repetitive bending stresses of high magnitude (*A*). Fatigue failure of the metal plate may occur (*B*).

shaft fragment is short or when there is comminution of the fragment, particularly laterally. Also, fixation may be difficult because the intramedullary canal is wide in the trochanteric area. The nail frequently cannot control rotation of the distal femoral shaft. In 1964, Zickel[65–67] developed a nail which purported to solve these problems. This device controls varus-valgus angulation due to bending by adding a cervical nail and by allowing controlled collapse of the segments due to axial compression even when there is medial comminution (Fig. 2.24). In addition, the rectangular cross section and contoured shape of the intramedullary rod controls rotation to some degree, and the proximal part of the rod is wide to fit the medullary canal in the trochanteric region.

In conclusion, subtrochanteric fractures of the femur are difficult to manage because high stresses in the subtrochanteric area make major demands on fixation devices. The frequent comminution of the medial cortical buttress complicates this fracture, and the method of treatment of the fixation device must deal with this complication. Controversy continues with regard to the best method of treatment of this problem fracture.

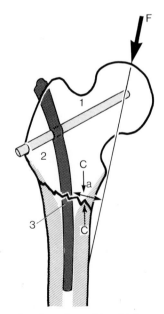

Figure 2.24. The biomechanics of combined intramedullary and cervical nailing. Controlled collapse of the fracture (axial compression, *c*) is possible around the intramedullary nail so that bony contact between the segments is maintained (*2*). Bending is resisted by the cervical nail (*1*). Bending stress on the implant is reduced owing to the short bending moment lever arm (*a*) (*3*). *F*, joint force.

KNEE JOINT

Knee Joint Biomechanics

As Morrison[42] has shown, the resultant joint force in the normal knee during walking is located primarily in the medial compartment. The magnitude of this force varies from individual to individual, but it is approximately three to four times body weight. The biomechanics of the knee, like that of the hip, can be discussed in terms of a first class lever system. The fulcrum is the point of bearing contact, i.e., the area of contact between the femoral and tibial bearing surfaces (Figs. 2.7 and 2.25). Body weight acting medial to the knee must be balanced by forces acting laterally. Like the hip, the knee is a first class lever "teeter-totter" system. At the hip, the abductor muscles balance body weight; at the knee it is the lateral soft tissues, i.e., lateral collateral ligament, fascia lata, and biceps femoris muscle. Because body weight acts medial to the knee joint, a moment is applied to the shank, which tends to adduct it relative to the thigh, i.e., to cause varus angulation. Because of this effect, the center of pressure (fulcrum) of the knee shifts to the medial side throughout most of the weight-bearing phase of the gait cycle. This is the normal biomechanical arrangement at the knee, but during normal gait and under certain pathological conditions, e.g., a paralytic limb with a Trendelenburg gait, the center of pressure may shift to the lateral compartment.[24] In this situation the shank is subjected to a moment which tends to abduct the tibia relative to the femur at the knee. To

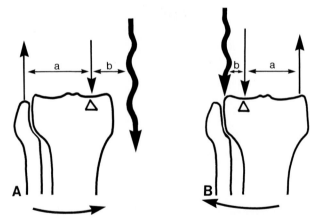

Figure 2.25.   A first class lever system at the knee. When the tibia is subjected to a bending moment which adducts the shank (*A*), a tension force occurs in the lateral ligament and a compression force over the medial tibial condyle. The reverse occurs when the knee is abducted (*B*).

achieve equilibrium, the medial collateral ligament is now placed under stress in conformity with the teeter-totter principle (Fig. 2.25).

Ligaments

It is possible, then, during weight bearing, for the shank to be adducted or abducted at the knee with the resultant joint force "C" centered over either the medial or lateral condyle. Equilibrium is achieved by forces in the collateral ligaments. The main function of the collateral ligaments is to resist abduction-adduction at the knee. In normal individuals, during ambulation the most common loading situation is the resultant joint force centered over the medial condyle and a tensile force in the lateral soft tissue structures. In addition to abduction-adduction moments, the knee is subjected to torsional loads during ambulation. Because the collateral ligaments are situated further from the center of the knee than the cruciates, they have a greater mechanical advantage for resisting abduction-adduction moments and torsional loads. Since they are located in the center of the knee, the cruciates are in a less mechanically advantageous position to resist either torque or bending. Their prime function is to prevent anteroposterior displacements of the tibia relative to the femur. A further biomechanical function of the cruciates is to resist hyperextension of the knee and the anterior cruciate is best suited for this purpose.

Menisci

The precise biomechanical role of the menisci is unknown, but presumably they act as shock absorbers. Their shapes are contoured to those of the femoral and tibial articular surfaces so that the menisci increase both knee-joint congruity and the area of contact, thereby distributing stress more uniformly across the bearing surface.[63] Because of their specific shape, they can act as anteroposterior and mediolateral stabilizers.

Muscles

The major muscle masses which span the knee joint are the quadriceps mechanism anteriorly, including the patella and patellar ligament and the hamstrings and gastrocnemii posteriorly. These muscles flex and extend the joint and stabilize it under weight-bearing conditions. The force of contraction for these muscles is frequently in the range of 300 to 500 lb, and their actions correspond to major peaks in knee-joint loading during walking.[24,42] For normal individuals, the joint force loads at the knee may be three to five times body weight. Presumably these loads are much higher during dynamic activity such as running and jumping. Impact loading, therefore, may produce a joint force at the knee which is many multiples of body weight (Fig. 2.26).

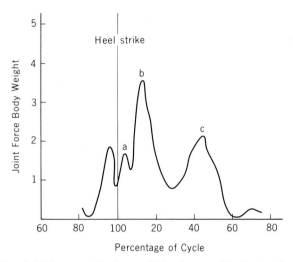

Figure 2.26.   Joint force at the knee. This diagram illustrates the major force peaks that occur during normal walking. Each peak corresponds to a major force action in particular muscle group. *a*, joint force peak due to hamstring muscle contraction; *b*, quadriceps contraction; *c*, gastrocnemius contraction.

Knee-Joint Injuries

During walking, the knee is normally subjected to the following types of load: abduction-adduction bending; axial compression; rotational torque; and shear forces acting parallel to the bearing surfaces.

Knee-joint injuries may be either to soft tissue or bone.

Soft Tissue Injuries

The most common mechanism of injury to the knee causing soft tissue damage is the combination of axial loading with abduction and external rotation moments. This can produce complete tearing of the medial collateral ligament including the posterior capsule, meniscal damage, and anterior-cruciate-ligament rupture (Fig. 2.27). This combination of medial collateral ligament and anterior cruciate and meniscal tearing is commonly known as the "terrible triad of O'Donoghue."[46] The reverse loading mechanism, i.e., axial loading combined with adduction and internal rotation moments, may damage lateral joint structures, i.e., lateral collateral ligament, lateral meniscus, and posterior cruciate. Kennedy et al. have accurately described these mechanisms[35, 36] and verified them experimentally on a cadaver stress machine.[34]

Pure flexion extension bending moments to the knee rarely cause injury, except that hyperextension can produce isolated tears of the

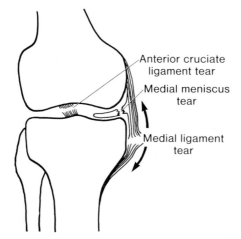

Anterior cruciate
ligament tear

Medial meniscus
tear

Medial ligament
tear

Figure 2.27.   Soft tissue injuries at the knee. Combined axial, abduction, and torsional loading may cause serious damage to the medial collateral ligament, including the posterior capsule, meniscus, and anterior cruciate ligament.

anterior cruciate ligament. The knee can be completely dislocated if enough force is applied, but fortunately this is an uncommon injury.

In recent years, classifications[31, 32, 41] of knee ligament injuries have varied from the simple anatomical approach of naming the major structures damaged to complex systems that emphasize the type of instability present (varus, valgus, anterior, posterior, translation, or rotation). To date, no single classification has won universal acceptance.

Whatever method is used to treat major ligament injuries of the knee involving both acute and chronic tears, the following principles are important:

Examination of an injured knee under general anesthesia is invaluable in assessing the degree of ligament damage, i.e., incomplete versus complete tears.

The knee should be examined in approximately 20° of flexion to relax the posterior capsular structures so as to permit proper assessment of collateral and cruciate ligaments. It should be noted that even though there are complete tears of all ligaments, if the posterior capsule is intact the knee may be stable when examined in extension.

Following surgical or conservative treatment of ligament injuries, the method of immobilization of the limb is important. For example, in medial ligament tears the limb should be immobilized in an above knee cast with the knee flexed to approximately 80° and the tibia internally rotated to relax the medial collateral ligament. This posture allows the ligament to heal in its shortest possible length, thereby enhancing stability.

Patellofemoral Joints

The patella functions as a sesamoid bone and gives mechanical advantage to the quadriceps tendon. The patella has a V shape on cross section and moves like a rope on a pulley in the intercondylar groove of the femur. The patella gives the quadriceps a mechanical advantage in flexing and extending the knee by increasing the lever moment arm from the center of rotation. Excision of the patella for disease or injury reduces the efficiency of this mechanism; hence, every attempt should be made to reconstruct the patella following injury. It is important to restore the patella's articular surface because high forces are transmitted across the patellofemoral articulation. Incongruity of the articular surface produces high stress concentrations on the joint surfaces and, in time, degenerative arthritis. The lever arm principle of the patella is illustrated in Fig. 2.28.

Bony Injuries of the Knee

As indicated earlier, the knee is subjected to abduction-adduction moments during normal walking. Trauma can increase these moments significantly so that the resultant joint force in either the medial or lateral condyle is increased above normal (pure adduction-abduction moments).

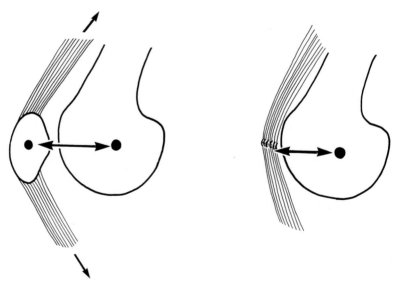

Figure 2.28. The biomechanics of the patella. Excision of the knee cap reduces the quadriceps-patellar ligament lever arm so that increased muscle force is required to extend the knee.

Under this abnormal loading, the ligaments may rupture or they may remain intact and contribute to femoral condyle or tibial plateau fractures. Here the mechanism of fracture is a combination of axial compression across the bearing surfaces, which may result in comminution and depression of the articular surface, combined with shear stresses which may split off the entire femoral or tibial condyle. Pure axial compression produces the Y or T condyle fracture, in which the femoral shaft impacts into the condyles, splitting them off. Again, this is an example of the first class lever system in action. The mechanism is similar to that of a nutcracker where the intact ligament acts as a hinge and the condyles are compressed. It is not clear why, under the same loading conditions, ligaments may rupture in one individual and condyles fracture in another, except that the type of damage is probably related to differing individual mechanical properties of ligament and bone. Osteoporosis for example, would produce a higher incidence of fractures than ligament ruptures, whereas ligament rupture is more likely in individuals with healthy bone.

The chief objectives in treating these fractures are to restore the congruity of the articular surfaces and secure the stabilized condylar fragments to the shaft in such a way as to prevent redisplacement.[43,56] The principle of the condylar and buttress plate has special significance in these bony injuries because in tibial plateau fractures it is important to secure the medial and lateral buttress in order to prevent late varus-valgus angulation deformity. Similarly, in the condylar region, fixation should prevent displacement of the condyle which would produce incongruity of the bearing surface and subsequent varus or valgus angular deformity[40] (Fig. 2.29 A and B).

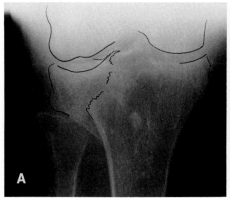 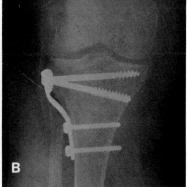

Figure 2.29. A and B, the buttressing of tibial plateau fractures. Following reduction, the buttress plate prevents redisplacement with subsequent angular deformity and joint incongruity. (The photographs illustrate before and after fixation of a tibial plateau fracture.)

Theoretically, the medial portion of the knee joint is most important for weight bearing since stress concentrations are highest here during walking.[24, 40, 42] It would seem important, then, to reconstitute the medial side as accurately as possible following fracture.

ANKLE JOINT

The biomechanics of the ankle joint have not been studied in as much detail as those of the hip and knee. During weight bearing the ankle is subjected to a small valgus moment in the frontal plane, which causes the lateral malleolus to function as a weight-bearing structure.[17, 43] Bolin[5] suggests that the lateral malleolus transmits up to one-sixth of body weight during ambulation. The medial malleolus is felt to be of less importance; working with the deltoid ligament, its main function seems to be to prevent eversion of the talus.

The articular surface of the talus is wider anteriorly than posteriorly, so that as the ankle is dorsiflexed the mortice widens. This happens because the anterior and posterior tibial fibular ligaments are elastic and the fibula is capable of some flexibility and torsion.[43, 56] Therefore, the ankle mortice, has a dynamic function. As the ankle is flexed and extended, the articular surface of the talus remains congruous with the tibial fibular mortice.

Loads transmitted by the ankle joint have not been accurately measured to date. However, simple mechanical analysis shows that standing on the toes of one foot can thrust a force of three times body weight across the ankle.[1] Unlike the hip and knee, where bearing surfaces are relatively large, the surface area of contact at the ankle is small, so that stress concentrations are high. Willenegger[43, 64] has suggested that small displacements of the talus, e.g., due to inaccurate reduction of the lateral malleolus, greatly reduces the area of weight-bearing surface of the talus. This change produces high stress concentrations during weight bearing and may encourage early arthritic change in the joint following fracture. He suggests that the most important criterion in assessing the results of ankle fractures is the development of early osteoarthritis. When no osteoarthritis develops, one may conclude that adequate biomechanical reduction had left no areas of abnormal cartilage pressure.

It would seem important, then, to obtain an accurate reduction following fracture of the ankle. The key to reduction is the lateral malleolus, since it has a weight-bearing function and controls the position of the talus. Several complex classifications of ankle joint fractures and dislocations have been suggested,[3, 39] but the simple classification offered here has been based on the mechanics of fracture. The key to understanding ankle fracture patterns lies in appreciating the biomechanics of the basic types of long bone fracture patterns (Ch. 1). In summary these are: 1) tension and bending loads produce a transverse fracture pattern, 2) torsion loads produce a spiral fracture pattern; and 3) axial compression results in joint compression or diaphyseal impaction fractures.

If these biomechanical principles are applied as the radiographs are analyzed, the surgeon will recognize the major forces producing most ankle fractures. There are three major fracture patterns:

Type I Abduction External Rotation Injuries

With this type of injury, the fibula (lateral malleolus) fractures at or above the level of the syndesmosis. The deltoid ligament or medial malleolus is frequently torn or avulsed. If the medial malleolus fractures, the break is of the transverse (avulsion) variety. In the commonest and simplest type, an isolated external rotation fracture of the lateral malleolus leaves the medial malleolus and the tibial fibular joints intact (Fig. 2.30 *A-C*). The spiral fracture of the fibula runs obliquely from anterior distally to posteriorly proximally; the fracture begins at the joint line, indicating that the syndesmosis has not been disrupted.

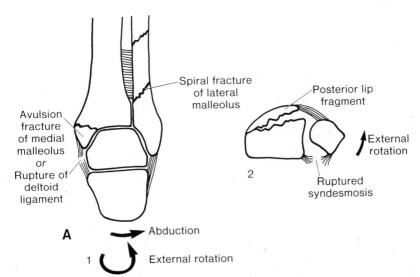

Figure 2.30. *A*, type I abduction external rotation injury of the ankle (*1*). Fracture of the lateral malleolus begins at or above the talar tibial joint lines. Avulsion fracture of the medial malleolus or deltoid ligament rupture occurs. When the lateral malleolar fracture occurs above the joint line, rupture of the anterior fibers of the syndosmosis occurs (*2*). The posterior syndosmosis remains intact and attached to the lateral malleolus and posterior tibial lip fragment. Anatomical reduction of the lateral malleolus almost invariably reduces the posterior lip fragment. The lateral malleolus is the key to reduction for this fracture type.

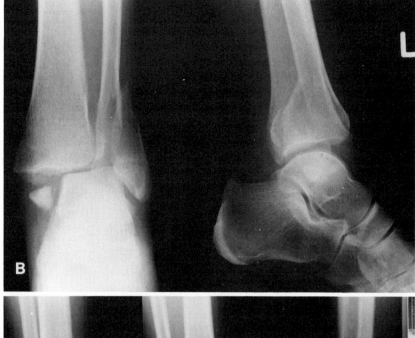

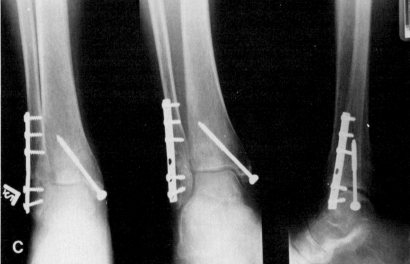

Figure 2.30.   *B* and *C*, illustrating before and after surgical correction of a type I fracture where the lateral malleolus fracture begins at the joint line and there is avulsion of the medial malleolus.

The higher the fracture, the greater the damage to the tibiofibular ligaments (syndesmosis); this pattern suggests that external rotation produced the injury. The anterior portion of the syndesmosis is frequently torn, and sometimes there is an associated avulsion fracture of the anterior edge of the lateral malleolus. With subsequent external rotation, the fibula is rotated outwards, tearing the anterior portion of the syndesmosis. Usually the posterior ligament, which is attached to the posterior lip of the tibia, remains intact and avulses the posterior lip of the tibia (the third malleolus). Isolated diastasis of the mortice is rare. The surgeon must look for a proximal fracture of the fibula which frequently indicates a more serious injury than simple fracture of the fibula, i.e., an external rotation injury with rupture of the deltoid ligament, tearing of the syndesmosis, and fracture of the proximal fibula (Fig. 2.30 *D* and *E*).

Treatment (Fig. 2.31)

Surgical treatment of the type I injury is directed to the lateral malleolus—to its accurate reduction and to the restoration of fibular length. Once this has been accomplished, the third malleolus is almost invariably reduced. Fixation of the medial part of the ankle is then undertaken. Diastasis is corrected with a transverse horizontal diastasis screw (to keep the mortice reduced while the ligaments heal). The screw must not produce compression because this may interfere with the inferior tibiofibular joint. The screw should be removed before weight bearing, usually at 6 or 7 weeks; if not, it will fracture.

Type II Adduction Internal Rotation Injuries (Injuries Below the Tibiofibular Joint)

With this type of fracture, the lateral malleolus is not the key to reduction. Fractures involving this structure occur at or below the tibiofibular joint and are pure avulsion injuries (Fig. 2.32 *A-C*). The fracture line involving the fibula is usually horizontal. The simplest injury of this type, the complete lateral ligament tear from an inversion injury, may be associated with a fracture of the medial malleolus. When the medial malleolus is fractured, the fracture line is frequently oblique or vertical, indicating a shearing injury from impaction of the talus against the medial part of the mortice. Posterior lip fractures may occur in combination with a fracture of the medial malleolus or separately, but they have no relationship to the syndesmosis or the fibula. Reduction of the fibula will not reduce the posterior lip fragments; these must be dealt with separately, It is important to emphasize that this type of fracture does not involve the syndesmosis, so that there is no threat of diastasis (separation of the ankle mortice).

Type III Fractures—Vertical Compression of Crush Injuries

In this situation, loading is axial and produces crushing of the articular surface of the lower tibia and considerable comminution. These fractures

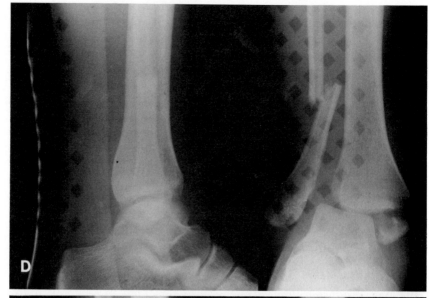

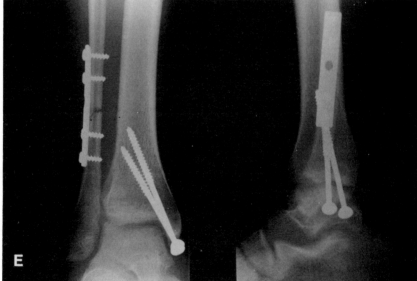

Figure 2.30. *D* and *E*, illustrating a type I fracture where the lateral fracture occurs above the joint line and there is complete disruption of the syndosmosis between the lower fibula and tibia.

are difficult to treat by internal fixation because of the multiplicity of fragments. Their prognosis is poor and the likelihood of degenerative change is greatly increased.

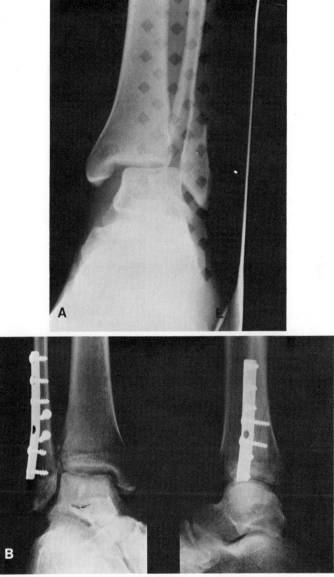

Figure 2.31.   *A*, a type I fracture of the lateral malleolus and avulsion of the deltoid ligament. There is significant lateral displacement of the talus. *B*, the fibula out to length and securely fixed. The deltoid ligament has been repaired and the ankle mortice is intact.

UPPER EXTREMITY INJURIES

The joints most frequently injured in the upper extremity are the shoulder, elbow, and wrist. In most instances the mechanism of injury is

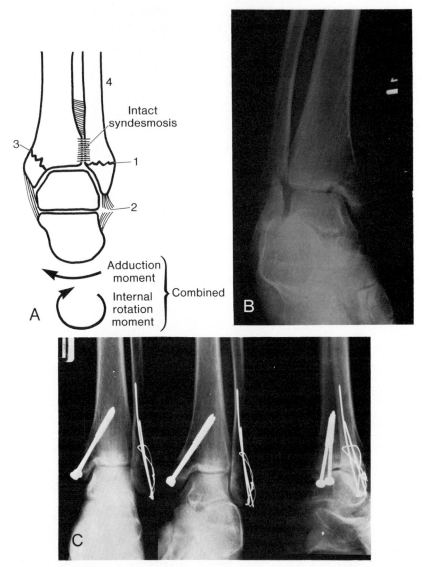

Figure 2.32.   *A*, type II adduction internal rotation injury of the ankle: *1*, horizontal avulsion type fracture of the lateral malleolus; *2*, lateral ligament rupture; *3*, oblique (almost vertical) fracture of the medial malleolus; *4*, intact syndesmosis. *B* and *C*, a type II fracture before and after surgical fixation.

a fall on the outstretched hand (Fig. 2.33). Mechanically, the upper extremity acts as a strut transmitting force from its point of contact with the ground (the hand) to the torso.[4] A weak strut gives way. Age,

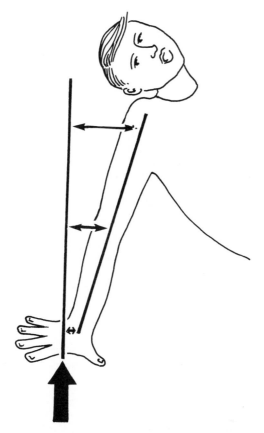

Figure 2.33. A fall on the outstretched hand produces a bending moment relative to the wrist, elbow, and shoulder. This may cause abduction-adduction or flexion extension bending at these joints, depending on the direction of the ground to hand force.

therefore, has a major influence on the type of injury. In the elderly, bone is usually weaker than ligaments; hence, fractures are more common toward the end of life, whereas dislocations are most frequent in the young. When an individual falls on the outstretched arm, force is transmitted along the strut until a weak point is reached. Colles' fractures are more common in the elderly since the force of impact is often dissipated at the first weak point in the strut, i.e., the wrist; in strong, young extremities, force is more apt to reach the base of the arm.

As Figure 2.34 illustrates, a fall on the outstretched arm will have two major mechanical effects: an axial compression force and a bending moment.

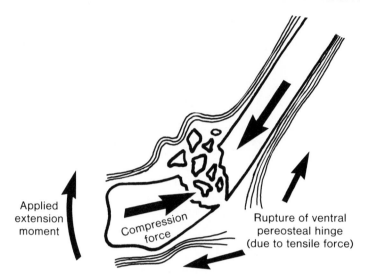

Applied extension moment

Compression force

Rupture of ventral pereosteal hinge (due to tensile force)

Figure 2.34. Colles fracture of the wrist. This fracture is due to the combination of an extension moment at the wrist and axial compression. Compression forces crush the dorsal cortex and tensile forces disrupt the ventral pereosteal hinge.

Analysis of the mechanism of injury must also consider torsion about the long axis of the strut (upper extremity) due to twisting of the arm during a fall.

Wrist

In adults, the most common injury at the wrist is the Colles' fracture, but a variety of injuries is possible, including carpal fractures, subluxation, and dislocation, and in children, epiphyseal displacement. The Colles' fracture has many interesting mechanical features, and since it is so common, it merits some discussion.

A fall on the outstretched hand causes axial compression combined with a bending moment which tends to dorsiflex the wrist. The net effect is a force couple which tends to compress the wrist dorsally while stretching the soft tissues on the ventral aspect (Fig. 2.34). Typically there is dorsal displacement of the distal radius associated with comminution of the dorsal cortex. Displacement ruptures the tissues on the volar aspect of the wrist but the tissues dorsally remain intact, forming a soft tissue hinge. Charnley[7] suggests that this hinge is the key to reduction of the fracture. When comminution is extensive, the fracture is unstable and may be difficult to control by casting. The instability is due to the dorsal comminution which allows the fracture to collapse (Fig. 2.34). Usually Colles' fractures can be controlled in a short arm cast or dorsal slab, using the three-point fixation principle described by Charnley. The key to success is to keep the soft tissue hinge under tension, as illustrated in Figure 2.35. Most Colles' fractures can be treated in this manner; however, when comminution is extensive and the fracture is very unstable, external skeletal fixation using an Anderson[2] apparatus is helpful (Fig. 2.36). This apparatus acts as an "outrigger," preventing collapse of the fracture and consequent recurrence of deformity.

Elbow

Injuries to the elbow are common during a fall on the outstretched hand. The type of injury is determined by the anatomy of the elbow and the nature of the applied load.

Anatomy

The lower end of the humerus can be viewed as two columns, one medial and one lateral. The lateral column has a small bearing surface which articulates with the proximal end of the radius (radial head). The medial column has a large bearing surface (trochlea) which articulates with the similunar notch of the ulna. The extensor muscles originate from the lateral epicondyle and the flexors from the medial epicondyle. Anteriorly, the biceps and brachialis flex the elbow, whereas the triceps, acting posteriorly, extend the joint. The elbow is stabilized by medial and lateral collateral ligaments.

In flexion, the elbow functions as a third class lever; i.e., the applied force (brachialis and biceps) acts between the fulcrum and weight. In

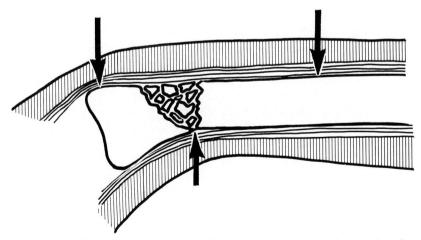

Figure 2.35. Three point pressure: Cast is molded to produce a bending moment that counters the one which originally created the fracture, thereby maintaining the reduction.

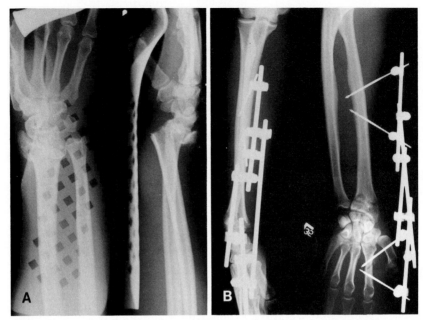

Figure 2.36. *A* and *B*, a comminuted Colles fracture before and after using the Roger Anderson apparatus for fixation. Unstable comminuted Colles fractures may require external skeletal fixation, such as that provided by this apparatus, to keep the fracture out to length and to maintain reduction.

extension, this joint functions as a first class lever; it has a low mechanical advantage because of the short lever arm from the triceps insertion to the center of rotation of the joint.

When an individual falls on the outstretched hand, three types of loading can develop at the elbow, singly or in combination (Fig. 2.37).

Hyperextension. The elbow may be forcibly extended. In this situation the proximal ulna impacts into the olecranon fossa, creating an extension bending moment at the elbow. In effect, the proximal ulna grips the lower end of the humerus like a vice, fracturing it in the supracondylar area where the bone is weak. This fracture is more frequent in children and is thought to occur because in the young the ligaments are stronger than bone so that force is transmitted across the elbow to the supracondylar region. With this injury, the soft tissue structures, i.e., periosteum at the front of the elbow, are torn, while the posterior tissues (posterior hinge) remain intact. Following reduction of the fracture, flexion of the elbow tightens the posterior hinge, stabilizing the fracture. Flexion of the forearm produces a stabilizing force couple; the fracture surfaces are compressed anteriorly and the posterior capsule is stretched

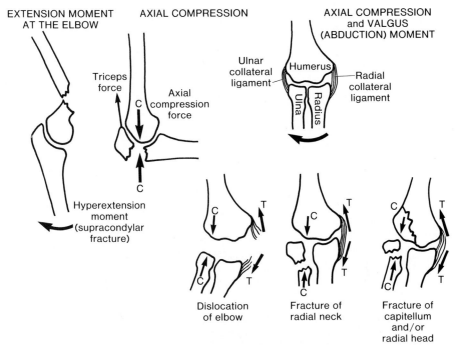

EXTENSION MOMENT
AT THE ELBOW

AXIAL COMPRESSION

AXIAL COMPRESSION
and VALGUS
(ABDUCTION) MOMENT

Triceps
force

Axial
C compression
force

Ulnar
collateral
ligament

Humerus

Radial
collateral
ligament

Ulna

Radius

C

Hyperextension
moment
(supracondylar
fracture)

Dislocation
of elbow

Fracture of
radial neck

Fracture of
capitellum
and/or
radial head

Figure 2.37.   Basic mechanics of elbow injuries. An extension moment applied
to the elbow will likely cause a supracondylar fracture. Axial compression (C)
may fracture either the olecranon or the humeral condyles (Y and T). Axial
compression combined with an abduction moment can cause fracture of the
capitellum due to a force couple which produces compression laterally and
tension (T) in the medial collateral ligament. The same mechanism can produce
fracture either of the radial head or radial neck. If the medial ligament ruptures,
dislocation or subluxation of the joint occurs.

posteriorly (Fig. 2.38). Because of the tendency for this fracture to develop
a cubitus varus "gun stalk" deformity, much attention has been paid to
the position of the forearm following reduction. Agreement has not been
reached as to whether the forearm should be immobilized in neutral,
pronation, or supination, but, from a mechanical aspect, the method of
Salter seems most logical.[55] If the distal fragment is displaced postero-
medially, the lateral periosteal or soft tissue hinge has been torn. The
medial hinge is intact. Pronating the forearm will produce a force couple,
tightening the medial capsular structures and compressing the fracture
surfaces laterally. With posterolateral displacement of the distal fragments, the lateral soft tissue hinge is intact and the medial tissues are
disrupted. Supinating the forearm compresses the fracture surfaces me-

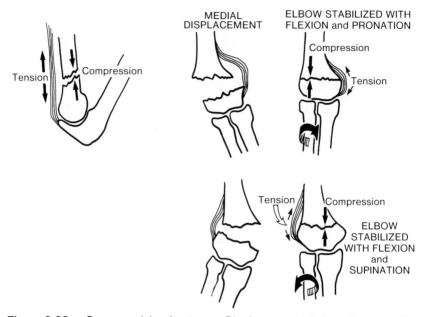

Figure 2.38. Supracondylar fractures. Displacement of the elbow medially indicates that the lateral hinge has been torn; therefore, flexion of the elbow and pronation of the forearm will tighten the posterior pereosteal hinge and the intact medial soft tissues, thereby maintaining the reduction. The reverse mechanics apply when initial displacement is posterolaterally.

dially while tensing the soft tissue structures laterally, as illustrated in Figure 2.38. Whether the forearm should be pronated or supinated can be determined from the displacement noted on the prereduction radiographs. It also should be recognized that a cubitus varus deformity may be secondary to internal rotation of the distal fragment.

Flexion type supracondylar fractures are rare and are usually due to a force applied to the posterior aspect of the distal humerus. The elbow, including the lower humerus, is displaced anteriorly. The mechanics of this injury are opposite to the more common extension type supracondylar fracture.

Axial Loading. A fall directly onto the elbow with the joint flexed applies an axial load to the shaft of the humerus. The force may split the articular surface of the humerus into two separate condyles (the Y or T-shaped fractures) or, more commonly, it may fracture the olecranon. When the condyles of the humerus split off, one or both of two fracture mechanisms may operate. The condyles may be separated by the splitting effect of the humeral shaft or by the wedging effect of the olecranon. The olecranon may be fractured by wedging by the distal humerus or by a violent triceps muscle contraction which avulses the olecranon process. In either situation (fractures of the distal humerus and olecranon) treatment is aimed at restoring the articular surfaces and maintaining the reduction so that early movement can prevent joint stiffness. Open reduction and internal fixation is frequently the method of choice.

Abduction-Adduction Loading. The most common mechanism of injury at the elbow is abduction combined with hyperextension loading. Theoretically, adduction injuries are possible but probably are rare.

Pure abduction or valgus loading may produce a number of combinations of injury in this first class lever system that has a considerable mechanical advantage. A fall on the outstretched hand applies force at some distance from the elbow, as an axial force and bending moment (Fig. 2.33). The moment (ground-to-hand force multiplied by its lever arm) must be resisted by the elbow structures. The fulcrum is the elbow and the resisting moment from a pure abduction load will be a force couple created by compression of the lateral articular surfaces and tension in the medial soft tissue-medial collateral ligament (Fig. 2.37).

With pure abduction loading, a number of injury combinations are possible: tearing of the medial ligament, as an isolated injury or associated with subluxation or posterolateral dislocation of the elbow; fracture of the radial head with the medial ligament remaining intact (fracture is produced by compression of the radial head against the capitellum); isolated fractures of the lateral condyle. In this situation the medial ligament and radial head remain intact but the lateral condyle is sheared off by the lateral compression force (nutcracker effect).

It is apparent that in these injuries, abduction stretches tissues on the medial side of the elbow, which in turn acts as a hinge. The lateral side of the joint is compressed, producing the injury previously described. Violent trauma may produce all of these injuries simultaneously, viz, fracture dislocation of the elbow. Treatment of all elbow injuries aims at the restoration of the congruity of articular surfaces and the stabilization of the joint so as to permit early movement. In fracture dislocation where comminution of the radial head necessitates excision, it may be difficult to achieve stability. In this situation, a radial head prosthesis may be inserted to stabilize the joint (Fig. 2.39 *A* and *B*).

Shoulder Injuries

Compared to the hip, the shoulder is unstable. Both are ball-and-socket joints but the shoulder has a very shallow cup. Here stability has been sacrificed for increased motion. Most movements at the shoulder occur between the head of the humerus and the glenoid. Stability is provided by the capsule, glenoid labrum, and shoulder girdle muscles, the most

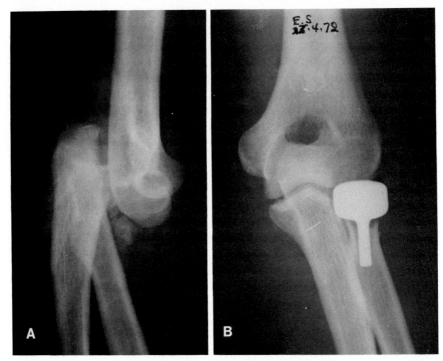

Figure 2.39. *A* and *B*, dislocation of the elbow associated with a comminuted fracture of the radial head is a serious injury. Excision of the head frequently results in an unstable joint. A radial head prosthesis acts as a "spacer" and stabilizes the joint.

important of which are the powerful deltoid, and the rotator cuff composed of the supraspinatus, infraspinatus, teres minor, and subscapularis. For stability, the humeral head must be kept closely applied to the glenoid so that it is unable to slip when a force is applied in any direction. The rotator cuff performs this function. When the arm hangs at the side, for example, contraction of the deltoid alone pulls the humeral head vertically. Contraction of the cuff muscle pulls the head against the glenoid, allowing the powerful deltoid to abduct the arm. The shoulder works as a third class lever with the head as the fulcrum.[4] The applied force (deltoid) acts between the fulcrum and the weight to be lifted. The rotator cuff keeps the humeral head applied to the glenoid, so that the shoulder can function efficiently as a third class lever (Fig. 2.40). When the cuff is torn, the humeral head is pulled upwards under the acromium, thereby reducing the leverage, viz, the deltoid lever arm is shortened.

As indicated earlier, the upper extremity acts a a strut in transmitting force from a fall on the outstretched hand. The position of the arm when

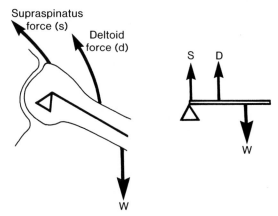

Figure 2.40. The shoulder functions as a third class lever. Forces which elevate the arm (deltoid muscle and rotator cuff) act between the fulcrum (shoulder joint) and the object to be lifted.

it conducts force to the shoulder does much to determine the type of shoulder injury. When the arm is adducted, the head of the humerus moves upwards against the coracoacromio arch, and the rotator cuff or acromium may be damaged rather than the clavicle. With the arm partially abducted, force is transmitted to the clavicle, fracturing this structure. When the arm is fully abducted (and externally rotated), maximum force is applied to the anteroinferior joint capsule and frequently produces anterior dislocation of the shoulder. This injury is commoner in younger patients where the rupture strength of capsule and ligaments is less than the fracture strength of bone. In the elderly, fracture of the shoulder is more common. Neer[44, 45] has classified shoulder fractures into two-part, three-part, and four-part injuries. The position of the humeral head following injury will depend on whether the tuberosities are intact. For example, disruption or avulsion of the greater tuberosity in the presence of an intact lesser tuberosity will rotate the articular surface of the humeral head posteriorly in response to the unopposed action of the subscapularis muscle. Conversely, an intact greater tuberosity in the presence of an avulsed lesser will result in an abducted, externally rotated position of the head fragments (Fig. 2.41). (The interested reader should refer to the paper in which Neer discusses the diagnosis and management of these shoulder injuries.) The most common complication of shoulder fractures is joint stiffness; hence, whatever method of treatment is used, conservative or surgical, early mobilization is essential to prevent stiffness.

As a rule, two-part fractures, where there is minimal displacement, can be treated conservatively. Three-part fractures are often treated by open

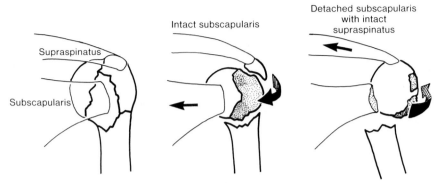

Figure 2.41. Shoulder fractures. In an intact subscapularis, the articular surface of the head of the humerus rotates posteriorly; in a detached subscapularis with an intact supraspinatus, the surface rotates anterolaterally.

reduction and internal fixation to secure the fragment in a reasonably accurate anatomical position. Four-part fractures are frequently associated with avascular necrosis of the humeral head due to the detachment of soft tissues. For this fracture Neer suggests replacing the articular segment with a prosthesis.

This chapter shows how the physician can apply basic mechanical concepts to the assessment and management of joint injuries. An understanding of the simple lever system enables him to appreciate the mechanics of joint loading in both abnormal and normal situations. Levers are classified according to the point of application of the applied force, the position of the fulcrum, and the object to be moved. Generally the first class lever, where the fulcrum is located between the applied force and object, is used to gain mechanical advantage. It is the prime lever system at weight-bearing joints such as the hip, knee, and ankle. At these joints body weight is balanced over a fulcrum (joint bearing surface) by forces acting in muscles and ligaments. Because of the "leverage effect," joint force is a multiple of body weight. Under abnormal conditions, such as impact loading from trauma, joint force may increase dramatically.

Injuries to the hip joint are common, and for this reason it is important to understand the biomechanical principles underlying their surgical treatment. The discussion of the mechanics of implant device fixation makes specific reference to subcapital, intertrochanteric, and subtrochanteric fractures. Shear, for example, is the major displacing force in subcapital fractures and successful management depends on an appreciation of its effect in terms of stability. The impacted, valgus Pauwels type I fracture is best suited to resist shear and is therefore stable; type III fractures resist shear poorly owing to the vertical fracture and are therefore unstable. At the intertrochanteric and subtrochanteric levels, the most significant problem is bending at the fracture site due to the applied joint force. Bending (bending moment) produces compression stresses in the medial cortex and tensile stress laterally. In both fracture types comminution of the medial cortex is common and tends to render then unstable. If comminution and the resulting defect in the medial buttress are ignored, excessive stress due to repetitive bending loads may produce fatigue failure of the metallic implant, nonunion or both. Regardless of the type of device used or its method of application, management always involves a race between fracture healing and implant failure. It is not possible to design a fail proof implant that is capable of resisting all conceivable loading situations. It is possible, however, to apply a knowledge of biomechanics to the treatment of hip fractures so that the bone rather than the device takes a major portion of the load. Medial displacement osteotomy, low angle nail insertion, and controlled collapse of fractures are examples of surgical methods that are based on biomechanical principles which minimize implant stress and facilitate fracture healing.

The knee has little intrinsic stability and depends on strong ligaments and muscles for support. These soft tissue structures transmit load across the joint and, owing to the leverage effect, bearing force is a multiple of body weight (three to five times body weight under normal circumstances). Abnormal loading can significantly increase joint and ligament force and produce ligament rupture or condyle fracture. It is important to restore congruity to the weight-bearing articular surfaces to prevent late degenerative changes. The medial side of the knee normally takes the major proportion of joint force, and this should be considered during surgical reconstructions.

The chapter provides a simple classification for ankle fractures based on the biomechanics of fracture. The lateral malleolus is the key to understanding the mechanics of injury and the rationale of treatment because it functions as a major weight-bearing structure and controls the ankle mortice. Small discrepancies in ankle mortice congruity may produce stress peaks and premature degenerative change due to a reduced area of bearing contact.

The lever system again operates in injuries involving the upper extremity and an understanding of basic mechanical concepts is essential for clarifying cause and treatment. Like those involving the lower limb, biomechanical techniques permit the surgeon to manage these injuries with greater understanding and confidence.

References

1. ALMS M: Fracture mechanics. *J Bone Joint Surg* 43B:162–166, 1961.
2. ANDERSON R, O'NEIL G: Comminuted fractures of the distal end of the radius. *Surg Gynecol Obstet* 78:434–440, 1944.

3. ASHHURST A, BROMER R: Classification and mechanism of fractures of the leg bones involving the ankle. *Arch Surg* 4:51–129, 1922.

4. BATEMAN JE: *The Shoulder and Environs.* CV Mosby, St. Louis, 1955.

5. BOLIN H: The fibula and its relationship to the tibia and talus in injuries of the ankle due to forced external rotation. *Acta Radiol (Stockh)* 56:439–448, 1961.

6. BRANTIGAN OC, VOSHELL AF: The mechanics of the ligaments and menisci of the knee joint. *J Bone Joint Surg* 23:44–66, 1941.

7. CHARNLEY J: *The Closed Treatment of Common Fractures,* ed. 3. E & S Livingston, Edinburgh, 1968.

8. COLLADO F, VILA J, BELTRAN JE: Condylocephalic nail fixation for trochanteric fractures of the femur. *J Bone Joint Surg* 55B:774–779, 1973.

9. DIMON JH III, HUGHSTON JC: Unstable intertrochanteric fractures of the hip. *J Bone Joint Surg* 49A:440–450, 1967.

10. DIMON JH III, HUGHSTON JC: Unstable intertrochanteric fractures. *Am Acad Orthop Surg Inst Course Lect* 19:110–118, 1970.

11. ENDER HG, BRIOT B: Per- and subtrochanteric fractures treated with Ender's flexible intramedullary pins. *Orthopaedic Transactions (JBJS)* 1:163–164, 1977.

12. EVANS EM: The treatment of trochanteric fractures of the femur. *J Bone Joint Surg* 31-B:190–203, 1949.

13. FIELDING JW: Subtrochanteric fractures. *Clin Orthop* 92:86–99, 1973.

14. FRANKEL VH: Mechanical principles for internal fixation of the femoral neck. *Acta Chir Scand* 117:427–432, 1959.

15. FRANKEL VH, BURSTEIN AH: *Orthopedic Biomechanics.* p 85, Lea & Febiger, Philadelphia 1970.

16. FRANKEL VH, BURSTEIN AH, BROOKS DB: Biomechanics of internal derangement of the knee. *J Bone Joint Surg [Am]* 53-A:945–962, 1971.

17. FRYER CM: Biomechanics of the lower extremity. *Am Acad Orthop Surg Inst Course Lect* 20:124–130, 1971.

18. GARDEN RS: The structure and function of the proximal end of the femur. *J Bone Joint Surg* 43-B:576–589, 1961.

19. GARDEN RS: Low-angle fixation in fractures of the femoral neck. *J Bone Joint Surg* 43-B:647–663, 1961.

20. GARDEN RS: Reduction and fixation of subcapital fractures of the femur. Symposium on fractures of the hip. Part II. *Orthop Clin Natl Am* 5:683–712, 1974.

21. HABOUSCH EJ: Photoelastic stress and strain analysis in cervical fractures of the femur. *Bull Hosp Joint Dis* 13:252–258, 1952.

22. HABOUSCH EJ: Biomechanics of femoral nail and nail plate insertions in fractures of the neck of the femur. *Bull Hosp Joint Dis* 14:125–137, 1953.

23. HABOUSCH EJ: A universal nail. Instruments for the treatment of fractures of the femur and biomechanical considerations. *Bull Hosp Joint Dis* 15:223–242, 1954.

24. HARRINGTON IJ: A bioengineering analysis of force actions at the knee in normal and pathological gait. *Bio-Med Eng* 11:167–172, 1976.

25. HARRINGTON KD, JOHNSON JO: The management of comminuted unstable intertrochanteric fractures. *J Bone Joint Surg* 55-A:1367–1376, 1973.

26. HELBIG FEJ, UNIS GL, FIELDING JW, WILSON HJ, RUBIN BD: A long-term end-result study of over one thousand intertrochanteric fractures. *J Bone Joint Surg* 59-B:504–505, 1977.

27. HOLT EP, JR: Hip fractures of the trochanteric region: treatment with a strong nail and early weight bearing. *J Bone Joint Surg* 45-A:687–705, 1963.

28. HOLT EP, JR: Unstable intertrochanteric fractures. *Am Acad Orthop Surg Inst Course Lect* 19:118–129, 1970.

29. HUGHSTON JC: Unstable intertrochanteric fractures of the hip. *J Bone Joint Surg* 46-A:1145, 1964.

30. HUGHSTON JC: Intertrochanteric fractures of the femur (hip). Symposium on fractures of the hip. Part I. *Orthop Clin N Am* 5:585–600, 1974.

31. HUGHSTON JC, ANDREWS JR, CROSS MJ, et al.: Classification of knee ligament instabilities. Part I & II. *J Bone Joint Surg* 58-A:159–179, 1976.

32. HUGHSTON JC, CROSS MI, ANDREWS JR: Classification of lateral ligament instability of the knee. 87th Annual Meeting of the American Orthopedic Association, San Francisco, 1975.

33. JACOBS NA, SKORECKI J, CHARNLEY J: Analysis of the vertical component of force in normal and pathological gait. *J Biomech* 5:11–34, 1972.

34. KENNEDY JC, FOWLER PJ: Medial and anterior instability of the knee. An anatomical and clinical study using stress machines. *J Bone Joint Surg* 53-A:1257–1270, 1971.

35. KENNEDY JC, GRAINGER RW: The posterior cruciate ligament. *J Trauma* 7:367–377, 1967.

36. KENNEDY JC, SWAN WJ: Lateral instability of the knee following lateral compartment injury. *J Bone Joint Surg* 54-B:763, 1972.

37. KOCH JC: The laws of bone architecture. *Am J Anat* 21:179–298, 1917.

38. KUNTSCHER G: A new method of treatment of pertrochanteric fractures. Part 1. *Proc R Soc Med* 63:1120–1121, 1970.

39. LAUGE-HANSEN N: Fractures of the ankle. IV. Clinical use of genetic roentgen diagnosis and genetic reduction. *Arch Surg* 64:488–500, 1952.

40. MAQUET PGJ: *Biomechanics of the Knee with Application to the Pathogenesis and the Surgical Treatment of Osteoarthritis.* Springer-Verlag, New York, 1976.

41. MARSHALL JL, RUBIN RM: Knee ligament injuries—a diagnostic and therapeutic approach. Symposium on injuries in sports: Recent developments. *Orthop Clin North Am* 8:641–668, 1977.

42. MORRISON JB: Bioengineering analysis of force actions transmitted by the knee joint. *Bio Med Eng* 4:164–170, 1968.

43. MULLER ME, ALLGOWER M, WILLENEGGFER H: *Technique of Internal Fixation of Fractures.* Springer-Verlag, New York, 1965.

44. NEER CS II: Displaced proximal humeral fractures. Part I. Classification and evaluation. *J Bone Joint Surg* 52-A:1077–1089, 1970.

45. NEER CS II: Displaced proximal humeral fractures. Part II. Treatment of three-part and four-part displacement. *J Bone Joint Surg* 52-A:1090–1103, 1970.

46. O'DONOGHUE DH: Surgical treatment of fresh injuries to the major ligaments of the knee. *J Bone Joint Surg* 32-A:721–738, 1950.

47. PAUL JP: Bioengineering studies of forces transmitted by joints—Part 2, Engineering analysis. In *Biomechanics and Related Bioengineering Topics,* edited by RM Kenedi. Pergamon Press, London, 1965.

48. PAUL JP: Biomechanics of the hip joint and its clinical relevance. *Proc R Soc Med* 59: 943–948, 1966.

49. PAUL JP: Forces transmitted by joints in the human body. *Proc Inst Mech Eng* 181:8–15, 1967.

50. PAUL JP: Magnitude of forces transmitted at hip and knee joints. In *Lubrication and Wear in Joints* edited by V. Wright, ch. 9. Sector Publishing Ltd., London, 1969, pp 77–87.

51. PAUL JP: Load actions on the human femur in walking and some resultant stresses. *Exp Mech* 11:121–125, 1975.

52. PAUWELS F: *Der Schenkelhalsbruch. Ein Mechanisches Problem. Grundlagen des Heilungsvorganges. Prognose un kausale Therapie.* Enke, Stuttgart, 1935.

53. PAUWELS F: The place of osteotomy in the operative management of osteoarthritis of the hip. *Triangle* 8:196–209, 1968.

54. RYDELL NW: Forces acting on the femoral head prosthesis: a study on strain gauge prostheses in living persons. *Acta Orthop Scand* (Suppl) 88:1–132, 1966.

55. SALTER RB: *Textbook of Disorders and Injuries of the Musculoskeletal System.* Williams & Wilkins, Baltimore, 1970.

56. SCHAUWECKER F: *The Practice of Osteosynthesis: A Manual of Accidental Surgery.* Chicago, Year Book Medical Publishers, 1974.

57. SCHUMPELICK W, JANTZEN PM: Die Versorgung der Frakturen im Trochanterbereich mit einer nichsperrenden Laschanschraube. *Chirurg* 24:506–509, 1953.

58. SCHUMPELICK W, JANTZEN, PM: A new principle in the operative treatment of trochanteric fractures of the femur. *J Bone Joint Surg* 37-A:693–698, 1955.

59. SEARS FW, SEAMANSKY MW: *University Physics,* ed. 2. Addison-Wesley Press, Cambridge, MA 1952.

60. SENN N: Fractures of the neck of the femur with special reference to bony union after intracapsular fractures. *Trans Am Surg Assoc* 1:333–452, 1883.

61. SMITH-PETERSEN MN, CAVE EF, VAN GORDER W: Intracapsular fracture of the neck of the femur. *Arch Surg* 23:715–759, 1931.

62. SMYTH EHJ, ELLIS JS, MANIFOLD MC, et al: Triangular pinning for fracture of the femoral neck. *J Bone Joint Surg* 46-B:664–673, 1964.

63. WALKER PS, HAJEK JV: The load bearing area of the knee joint. *J Biochem* 5:581–589, 1972.

64. WILLENEGGER H: Die Behandlung der Luxationsfrakturen des oberen Sprunggelenks nach biomechanischen Gesichtspunkten. *Helv Chir Acta* 28:225–239, 1961.

65. ZICKEL RE: A new fixation device for subtrochanteric fractures of the femur; a preliminary report. *Clin Orthop* 54:115–123, 1967.

66. ZICKEL RE: An intramedullary fixation device for the proximal part of the femur. *J Bone Joint Surg* 58-A:866–871, 1976.

67. ZICKEL RE, MOURADIAN WH: Intramedullary fixation of pathological fractures and lesions of the subtrochanteric region of the femur. *J Bone Joint Surg* 58-A:866–871, 1976.

Questions—Chapter 2

1. Shear force is most important for stability in:
   a. two-part intertrochanteric fractures
   b. subtrochanteric fractures
   c. subcapital fractures
   d. four-part intertrochanteric fractures

2. Stress on Ender's (intramedullary) nails is low because:
   a. the nails are designed to resist compression loading
   b. the nails have a relatively large cross-sectional area to resist shear stress
   c. the nails are closer to the line of action of the hip force so that bending stress on the implant is reduced
   d. they are better able to resist rotational loads

3. Normal loading of the femur causes maximum compression stress:
   a. along the calcar
   b. in the subcapital region
   c. in the intertrochanteric area
   d. in the subtrochanteric area

4. Comminution of the medial cortex with subtrochanteric fractures is significant because:
   a. the medial buttress is lost
   b. the area of contact between the main fracture fragments is reduced
   c. high tensile stresses occur in plate fixation devices so that metallic fatigue failure is frequent
   d. maximum bending stresses occur in the subtrochanteric region
   e. all of the above are true
   f. none of the above are true

5. Stability following reduction of a supracondylar fracture of the elbow depends on:
   a. the cast
   b. the intact periosteal hinge
   c. perfect reduction of the bony fragments
   d. pronation of the forearm

6. When initial displacement of an extension type supracondylar fracture is medially, stability is enhanced following reduction by:

    a. placing the forearm in supination
    b. placing the forearm in neutral position
    c. placing the forearm in pronation
    d. flexing the elbow

7.   In the first class lever system:
    a. the fulcrum is located between the force and the object to be moved
    b. there is greater mechanical advantage than for second and third class levers
    c. the mechanical advantage is increased by increasing the effort lever arm
    d. all of the above statements are true
    e. none of the above statements are true

8.   Abduction-external rotation injuries of the ankle are likely to cause:
    a. a transverse fracture of the lateral malleolus
    b. a spiral oblique fracture of the lateral malleolus below the level of the syndesmosis
    c. a spiral oblique fracture of the lateral malleolus at or above the syndesmosis
    d. an oblique fracture of the medial malleolus

9.   Adduction-internal rotation injuries of the ankle are likely to cause:
    a. a transverse fracture of the medial malleolus
    b. a spiral oblique fracture of the lateral malleolus
    c. a sprain or rupture of the lateral ligament of the ankle
    d. an oblique fracture of the medial malleolus, and/or a transverse lateral malleolus fracture at or below the joint line

10.   With abduction-external rotation injuries of the ankle:
    a. there is a spiral oblique fracture of the lateral malleolus beginning at or above the joint line
    b. the syndesmosis is torn except for its posterior tibiofibular component, when a posterior malleolar fragment is present
    c. reduction of the lateral malleolus will invariably reduce the posterior malleolus
    d. there is frequently a tear of the deltoid ligament or a transverse avulsion fracture of the medial malleolus

11.   At the shoulder the rotator cuff functions:
        a. to increase the deltoid muscle lever arm
        b. to stabilize the head of the humerus against the glenoid
        c. to prevent upward migration of the humeral head
           against the undersurface of the acromion
        d. to provide a steady fulcrum for the deltoid so that it
           acts most efficiently
        e. as a component (effort force) of a third class level
           system

12.   A fall on the outstretched arm often produces an applied
        moment which tends to:
        a. produce dorsiflexion at the wrist
        b. abduct and extend the elbow
        c. abduct the shoulder
        d. cause an axial compression force at the wrist elbow
           and shoulder

CHAPTER 3

Biomechanics of Internal Fixation

Eric R. Gozna

Nowhere does a proper balance between understanding the principles of tissue healing and basic engineering become more important than in the subject of osteosynthesis.

During the past decade, orthopedic surgeons have witnessed a vast proliferation of commercial devices whose principal raison d'etre has been to achieve the ideal of "rigid internal fixation." Each season brings a new product line to supplant those currently in vogue and claiming to have mechanical properties superior to those of competitors. The never-ending search for the *ideal device* has focused attention away from the true cause of most failures of internal fixation—not the failure of the device itself but the failure of the surgeon to appreciate the basic mechanical principles underlying its use and hence the failure to carry out a proper osteosynthesis. Bearing this in mind, the following chapter has been written not as a compendium of currently available fixation devices but rather to outline a few of the basic underlying biomechanical principles involving the three most commonly used osteosynthesis devices: the orthopedic screw, the bone plate, and the intramedullary nail.

BIOMECHANICS OF SCREW FIXATION

The most common orthopedic implant is the screw. Though this humble unit in the orthopedic armamentarium generally is taken for granted, a great deal of engineering technology has contributed to its design.[2, 8, 9, 19, 20, 26, 36]

Mechanically, a screw may be thought of as a device for converting a torsional load into an axial compression load. This is illustrated in Figure 3.1. As the surgeon applies torsion to tighten it, the screw advances into the bone until the head strikes the cortex. Thereafter, further tightening results in increased compression between the head and the bone. The actual torque that is converted into axial compression is called the

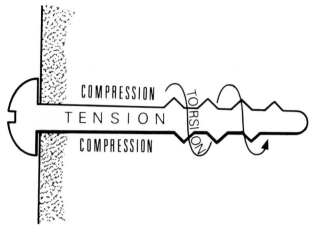

Figure 3.1.   Biomechanics of the screw.

"effective torque" and is the functional component. The two other ways that torsional energy can be expended are in overcoming thread friction and in cutting the thread.

The ideal design of screw and screw hole would maximize the amount of effective torque delivered and minimize the torsional energy expended in overcoming friction and cutting the thread.[19] This can be achieved most simply if the surgeon selects the proper design screw and proper diameter drill hole and pretaps the bone before insertion of the screw. However, the surgeon's knowledge should go beyond that. He should also appreciate some of the factors that go into the design of the various orthopedic screws and the indications for and contraindications to their use. Biomechanically, the humble orthopedic screw is truly a fascinating structure.

The screw consists of four parts: head, shaft, thread, and tip. There is an optimal design of each of these four parts in any specific orthopedic application.

Head

The head of a screw performs two functions. It acts as a couple between the screwdriver and the screw, and it provides the surface against which the compression force acts.

Figure 3.2 shows the four most popular screw head designs. Each has its particular attributes.

Slotted Head

This traditional design has a simple slot, is easy to manufacture, and can be removed with practically any standard screwdriver. However, it is

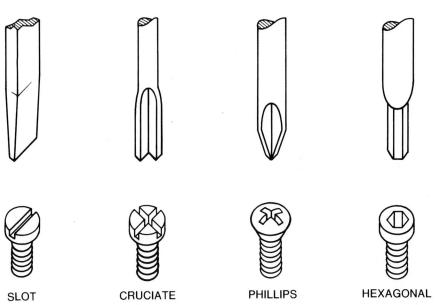

SLOT   CRUCIATE   PHILLIPS   HEXAGONAL

Figure 3.2. Four common designs of screw head.

the least efficient design because an illfitting or slightly malaligned screwdriver can slip off and burr the screw. This is called "caming out." For this reason the slotted screw is now being used less frequently.

Cruciate Head

The second slot at right angles to the first provides a much larger contact area between the screwdriver tip and the head, and hence reduces the tendency to "cam out." The disadvantage of this design is that the driver must be of the correct size to fit the screw and, since the screw and driver are not firmly coupled, the surgeon has little control over the screw's axial alignment.

Phillips Head

This self-centering device is easier to couple to the screwdriver. Otherwise it has little advantage over the cruciate head and has the theoretical disadvantage that the deep hole may induce corrosion because the oxygen tension is lower at its base.[10] For the modern low corrosion alloys, this is probably of little consequence.

Hexagonal Head

This is currently the most popular of head designs. It offers firm coupling with the driver, gives the surgeon much better control of screw alignment, and also has little tendency to "cam out."

As previously mentioned, in addition to serving as a couple between the screw and the driver, the head provides the surface against which the compression load is exerted. Depending on the head design, sufficient shear and bending forces may be set up at the junction of the head and the shaft to break the screw. Breakage can occur if the screw is not properly centered over the hole in a plate or if it is not inserted at right angles to the plate. The *spherically shaped head* is designed to reduce the shearing forces that are produced when a screw is not inserted at right angles with a plate. The self-compressing plate, to be described later in this chapter, utilizes eccentric placement of the screw to convert axial compression along the screw to tension along the plate and hence interfragmental compression (compression between the fracture fragments).

Shaft (Shank)

The shaft, or shank, is the smooth portion of the screw between the head and the thread, providing a link between the two. The thread is the active part of the screw, converting the applied torsional load into a tension load in the shaft (Fig. 3.1). The head, in turn, converts this tension load into a compression load as it advances toward and pushes against the cortex of the bone. The biomechanical importance of the shaft lies in its role as a mechanical link between the head and the thread.

The orthopedic surgeon selects a screw of a certain shaft length depending on the use for which the screw is intended. Though a number of screw designs are available for orthopedic purposes, they can all be classified into two categories according to their shaft length: those with short shafts are *machine screws*, while those with long shafts are *lag screws*. The indications for and the contraindications to these two types of screws will be elaborated upon in the sections to follow.

An understanding of the mechanics of the screw requires an appreciation of the principle of *lag fixation*. A concept that has only recently been appreciated by many orthopedists, lag fixation is the technique whereby a screw can produce compression between two objects (in fracture surgery this refers specifically to interfragmental compression). The conditions essential for interfragmental compression are: the screw thread must grip only the distal fragment, and the portion of the screw in the proximal fragment must be free to "glide" as the screw tightens. These conditions can be accomplished by using a lag screw or by using a machine screw and overdrilling the proximal fragment (producing a glide hole) (Fig. 3.3).

Since it is designed with a long shaft, the *lag screw* ensures that the portion in the proximal fragment is free to glide as the screw tightens. The most efficient shaft length for a lag screw is the shortest one which will allow the thread to be seated entirely in the distial fragment, thus achieving interfragmental compression.

As pointed out above, lag fixation can also be achieved using a standard maching screw if the surgeon "overdrills" the proximal fragment of bone. This creates a *glide hole*, which allows the proximal bone fragment to "glide" toward the distal one as the screw is tightened. To ensure that the screw threads do not engage in the proximal fragment, the glide hole must have a diameter equal to or greater than the thread diameter (widest diameter of the thread). It is impossible to achieve interfragmental compression with a cortical screw unless a glide hole is made before inserting the screw (Fig. 3.4).

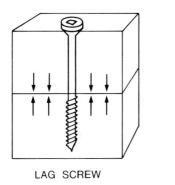

LAG SCREW

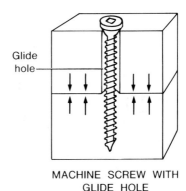

Glide hole

MACHINE SCREW WITH GLIDE HOLE

Figure 3.3.   Two ways of producing lag fixation.

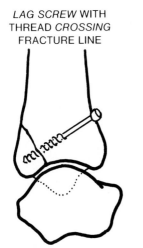

LAG SCREW WITH THREAD CROSSING FRACTURE LINE

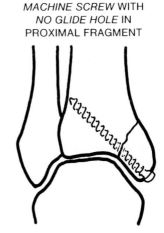

MACHINE SCREW WITH NO GLIDE HOLE IN PROXIMAL FRAGMENT

Figure 3.4.   Two common reasons for failure to achieve interfragmental compression using orthopedic screws.

Figure 3.5 shows a trimalleolar fracture of the ankle that was inade-
quately reduced and fixed with two machine screws. The medial malleolar
screw was inserted without creating a glide hole and a gap remained even
though the screw was tightened firmly (i.e., it created no interfragmental
compression). The lateral side was also not adequately reduced and fixed.
As one would anticipate, the reduction "slipped" within 2 months of the
surgery and subluxated into its original preoperative position. A second
operation was necessary, and this time the reduction was maintained by
using a figure-of-eight tension band to achieve good interfragmental
compression of the medial malleolar component and a "neutralization
plate" to maintain the fibular reduction. The fracture then healed uneventfully. If the surgeon had initially appreciated the need for adequate
reduction and internal fixation, and specifically the principle of lag
fixation, this failure might have been avoided.

Certain situations determine whether it is perferable to employ a lag
screw or a cortical screw with a glide hole:

Type of Bone

Because of the poor holding power of screws in cancellous bone
compared with cortical bone, large diameter threads are usually required.
To overdrill the proximal cortex and create a large diameter glide hole
would compromise the contact area between the screw head and the bone
cortex, unless a washer was used. In this situation the surgeon usually
will elect to use a lag screw rather than a wide diameter screw and glide
hole.

The Size of Proximal Fragment

If the fragment is small, it is generally wise to use a lag screw because
the proximal bone may break when the fragment is being overdrilled. Lag
screw fixation of medial malleolar fractures has become popular because
the tip of the malleolus is often small and the bone of the distal tibia is
cancellous. Because of its frequent use in this type of fracture, this
particular lag screw has become known as a "malleolar screw." Similarly,
the lag screw commonly used to reduce scaphoid fracture or nonunions
has become known as the "scaphoid screw." Screw fixation of scaphoid
fractures, as with malleolar fractures, usually involves dealing with relatively soft cancellous bone and small fragments. This situation lends itself
well to fixation with lag screws (Fig. 3.6).

Length of Time

The length of time the screw is expected to remain in the bone also
influences the choice of screw. If the screw is to be left in for a long time,

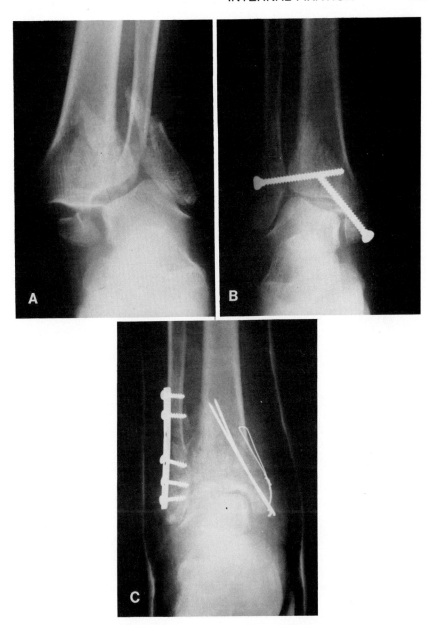

Figure 3.5.   Trimalleolar fracture of ankle with subluxation of talus. *B*, inadequate fixation of fracture with two cortical screws. Fracture is subluxated. *C*, reoperated upon. Adequate fixation with figure-of-eight tension band of medial malleolus with neutralization plate on lateral malleolus.

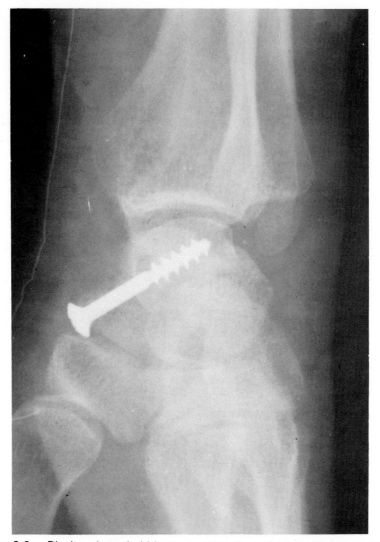

Figure 3.6.   Displaced scaphoid fractures are suited for internal fixation with a lag screw, because the fracture involves cancellous bone and the proximal pole is frequently small. This painful, displaced, ununited fracture was treated with just such a "scaphoid screw."

a machine screw is often preferred to prevent screw breakage upon removal. As the fracture unites, bone tends to grow around the shaft of the screw, obliterating the thread tract; this can make it impossible to remove the screw without breaking the screw off.

Securing a Plate

In the diaphyseal region, a machine screw is generally used for this purpose. Since compression is produced between the plate and the bone and most plates have a counter sink, only a short shaft is required. The other advantage of using the short shaft (machine) screw is that thread purchase is achieved in both the proximal and distal cortex. If a lag screw were used, only the distal cortex could be gripped by threads and the pull-out resistance would be greatly reduced.[5] The machine screw frequently used to secure plates in the diaphyseal region has become known as a "cortical" screw.

To secure a plate in the metaphyseal region one has to rely on the soft cancellous bone to resist pull-out (as the cortical bone is thin). In this situation one would select a screw with a wide thread diameter to give maximum pull-out resistance. This could be either a lag or a machine screw.

Thread

A screw works by virtue of the thread converting the torsional load into a compression load. Over the years the design of the orthopedic screw has evolved from that of a wood screw with a tapering thread, which augers its way through a material, to that of the highly sophisticated buttress thread machine screw. Considerable engineering technology has gone into the design of the orthopedic screw. The factors that must be considered in selecting the screw thread are: root diameter, thread diameter, lead, pitch, and root area of the tapped hole (Fig. 3.7).

The *root diameter* (also known as inside or core diameter) is the narrowest diameter of the screw. It is generally the weakest point of a screw. The smaller the root diameter, the greater the tendency to shear off during insertion, removal, or under various load conditions. The strength of a screw varies with the cube of its root diameter, hence a small change in root diameter markedly affects its strength.[2, 14] Though most screws fail because the pull out of the bone, approximately 10% of failures result from screw breakage. The usual point at which stress concentrates is the junction between the shaft and the thread.[2] This point, called the "run out," represents a sudden change in cross-sectional area and hence acts as a stress concentrator. Figure 3.8 shows a cortical screw that broke during removal from the bone. The characteristic location of the fracture is at the "run out," and the fracture has a spiral configuration indicating failure under a torsional load.

The *thread diameter* (outside diameter), the widest diameter of the thread, is one of the major factors affecting the screw's pull-out strength. The larger the outside diameter, the greater the resistance to pull-out.

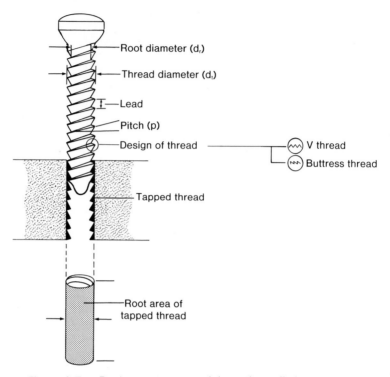

Figure 3.7.   Design parameters of the orthopedic bone screw.

This is the reason that most "cancellous" screws have a wide diameter thread.

The *pitch* is the distance between adjacent threads. A standard 4.5 mm cortical screw with approximately 15 threads per inch has a pitch of 0.07 inch. A screw with a fine thread has a small pitch and one with a coarse thread has a large pitch.

The *lead* is the distance a screw advances with each turn. For a single threaded screw, the lead equals the pitch (e.g., with each turn a 4.5 mm cortical screw will advance 0.07 inch). For a double threaded screw, the lead is twice the pitch (i.e., it advances twice as fast). Though a double threaded screw advances twice as fast as a single threaded screw, its mechanical advantage is less, so more torsional energy is required to produce the same amount of compression. For this reason, most orthopedic screws are single threaded. Mechanically, lead and pitch are analogous to the incline of a ramp; the steeper the incline, the shorter the distance a barrel will have to roll before it gets to the top, but the harder it is to push up the ramp.

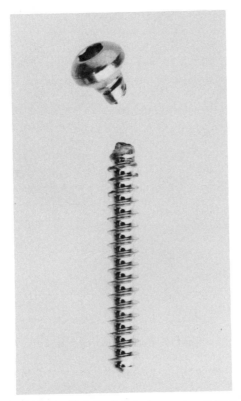

Figure 3.8.   Cortical screw that broke during removal from bone. Break occurred at characteristic location ("run off") between shaft and thread. The sudden change in shape produces stress concentration.

The *root area of the tapped thread* is an important determinant of the pull-out resistance of an orthopedic screw.[16, 19] As Figure 3.7 illustrates, if a traction force is applied to a screw, the bone at the tips of the thread is subjected to enormous shear forces. The concentration of the forces depends upon the thread diameter (d_T), the distance between the threads (pitch, p), and the length of the thread. Hence, the resistance to pull-out depends upon the area of bone at the tips of the threads or the root area of the tapped thread.

The *design* of a thread refers to its cross-sectional shape (Fig. 3.7). Two thread designs are commonly encountered in orthopedics: the buttress thread and the V thread. There is controversy as to which design has the greater pull-out strength.[9, 20] Theoretically, they should have the same pull-out strength if each has the some root area.[16] The proponents of the buttress type thread feel that its advantage lies not so much in its initial

THREAD DESIGN   ROOT AREA OF TAPPED THREAD

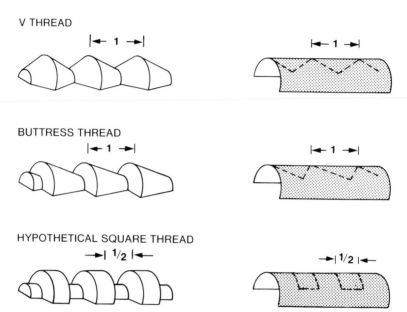

Figure 3.9.   Pull-out strength is determined by the root area of tapped thread (RATT). The hypothetical "square" thread has ½ the RATT of the "v" thread or buttress thread and hence only ½ the pull-out resistance. (Modified and reprinted with permission from V. H. Frankel and A. H. Burstein. *Orthopedic Biomechanics: The Application of Engineering to the Musculature System.* Lea & Febiger, Philadelphia, 1970.)

pull-out strength but in the improved strength that occurs after the screw has been left in situ for some time. This occurs through the ingrowth of bone around the thread (especially on its "buttress" aspect). Their argument is based on the premise that the buttress thread produces mainly compressive forces at the bone-thread junction, whereas the V thread produces both compression and shear forces. Since it is generally felt that bone resorption occurs in response to shear forces,[31,38] it has been proposed that the lower shear forces created by the buttress thread will result in less tendency towards screw loosening. To illustrate the effect of the buttress thread on bone remodeling, excellent diagrams of histological sections have been presented showing the increased bone deposition on the compression side of the buttress thread.[28]

Figure 3.9 shows several hypothetical designs of thread.[16] Recalling that the pull-out strength is reflected in the root area of the tapped thread, one would expect thread designs A and B to have the same pull-out strength, while C would have only half the pull-out resistance of the other two. This is because thread C has half the root area of the other two.

Tip

Three shapes of screw tips are commonly encountered in orthopedic surgery: fluted, rounded, and trocar (Fig. 3.10).

1. The *fluted* tip identifies the screw as being *self-tapping*. This screw creates its own thread as it advances into the bone. The main advantage of this screw is simplicity, as it requires no pretapping of the bone before insertion. This type of screw is mainly used in soft metaphyseal bone, where it can be inserted quickly and without difficulty. However, a non-self-tapping screw has certain advantages in hard, brittle cortical bone.

2. The non-self-tapping (or pretapped) screw had a *rounded* tip and a thread which extends to the tip. The rounded tip guides the screw easily into the pretapped hole. Before insertion of the screw, the hole has to be tapped with a special instrument. In recent years the tendency has been to convert to the non-self-tapping screw for orthopedic use, especially for screws used in cortical bone. In this situation the non-self-tapping screw has a number of advantages:

a. The taps are engineered to minimize heat production (by distributing the cutting area over many small surfaces) and to produce less microfracturing of the tapped cortical bone.[28] The result is a better constructed and stronger tapped thread in the bone.

b. The non-self-tapping screw can be removed and reinserted without scarring the thread.

c. The tip of the non-self-tapping screw has much greater resistance to pull-out than the fluted tip of the self-tapping screw, and hence tends to have a much better purchase on the distal bone cortex of the diaphyseal bone. Experimental evidence shows that the holding power of the fluted

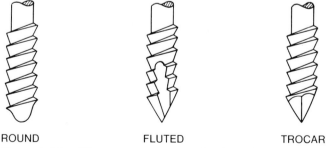

ROUND   FLUTED   TROCAR

Figure 3.10.   Three common types of orthopedic screw tips.

portion is approximately one-quarter that of a fully threaded portion of screw.[20]

d. The thread is tapped before the insertion of the screw, hence a greater "effective torque" can be produced when the scew is inserted. This results in a higher interfragmental compression.[26]

In spite of its disadvantages, the self-tapping screw still has considerable application in orthopedic surgery. Its main use is as a cancellous bone screw or where pull-out strength is not critical.

3. The *trocar* tip functions somewhat like a self-tapping screw. However, the trocar does not produce a true thread but rather displaces the bone as it advances. The "molleolar" screw has a trocar tip which is well suited for the soft cancellous bone of the distal tibia and medial molleolus.

In summary, when choosing an orthopedic screw, the surgeon should think in terms of its four components (head, shaft, thread, tip) and select the optimal screw for the particular application. For example, if it is anticipated that the scew will not be removed for quite some time or if the bone is hard, than the hexagonal *head* will ensure the best coupling between the screw and driver, lessening the tendency to "cam out" upon insertion or removal. If the proximal cortex is soft, then consider using a washer to increase the contact area between the screw head and the bone. The *shaft length* (i.e., choice between a lag or machine screw) is dictated by whether the surgeon wishes to achieve interfragment compression, the type of bone, and the size of the proximal bone fragment. To obtain interfragmented compression with a lag screw, the shaft length (nonthreaded portion) must be sufficient so that no thread extends across the fracture line when tightened. If a machine screw is used for this purpose a glide hole must be created in the proximal fragment. If the screw is used to secure a plate in the diaphyseal region, a short shaft length machine or "cortical" screw will give the greatest pull-out resistance, as it will purchase both the proximal and distal cortices.[5] The selection of the *thread shape* is not of great concern to the orthopedist, as virtually all of the commonly used orthopedic screws have been well engineered in this regard.[2,7] However, if the bone is soft (i.e., metaphyseal) and diminished pull-out strength is a potential problem, select a thread with a wide *outside diameter*. If screw breakage is the major concern, use a screw with a wide *root diameter*. Although the choice between self and non-self-tapping screws still remains a matter of personal choice or convenience with many surgeons, the orthopedist should at least be aware of the relative theoretical advantages of both types of screw. Probably the most common errors in regard to the use of the self and non-self-tapping screws is failure to recognize the difference at surgery. This can be quickly resolved by merely looking at the *tip*. If there is no fluted portion, one is dealing with a non-self-tapping screw designed to have the bone pretapped before insertion. An awareness of the above guidelines can avoid many needless frustrations in using the orthopedic screw.

SCREW FIXATION OF OBLIQUE FRACTURES

When the topic of screw fixation of oblique long bone fractures arises, a long discussion invariably ensues on the relative merits of inserting the screws at right angles to the fracture line, right angles to the shaft of the bone, or at some intermediate angle. Considerable biomechanical research has been done in an attempt to settle this matter.[3,5,24]

Figure 3.11, which summarizes the biomechanics of screw fixation of oblique long bone fractures, shows that for each load configuration

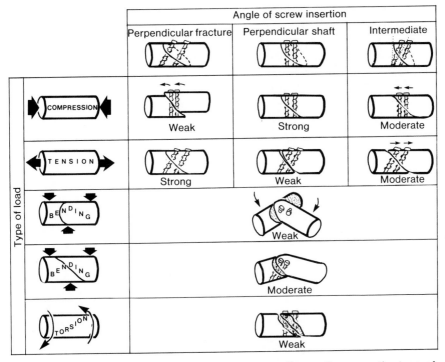

Figure 3.11.   Screw fixation of oblique fractures. Depending upon the type of *load*, various *angles of screw insertion* (perpendicular to fracture line, perpendicular to shaft, or intermediate angle) will confer different degrees of stability. (Modified and reprinted with permission from V. H. Frankel and A. H. Burstein. *Orthopedic Biomechanics: The Application of Engineering to the Musculature System.* Lea & Febiger, Philadelphia, 1970.)

(compression, tension, bending, or torsion) a certain angle of screw insertion produces maximum rigidity.[16] However, no single screw insertion angle provides excellent rigidity against all load configurations. For example, fixation with the screws at right angles to the plane of the fracture line provides good stability against tension loads but is less stable against compression loads. In contrast, screws inserted at right angles to the shaft provide stability against compression loads but not tension loads.[16] Since most long bones (especially those of the lower extremity) are intermittently subjected to both tension and compression loads, neither of the above insertion angles provides ideal fixation. One solution is to insert the screw at an angle intermediate to the angle perpendicular to the shaft and perpendicular to that of the fracture line (Fig. 3.12A). Another alternative for the long oblique or butterfly fracture is to insert several screws at right angles to the shaft for axial loading stability and several at a combined angle for combined interfragmental compression and tension loading[28] (Fig. 3.12B). Both techniques have their advocates. However, the most important point for the surgeon to determine is which loads predominate for a particular long bone or fracture configuration and then to insert the screws at an angle which will confer maximum stability against these loads. This approach requires first defining the "personality" of the fracture and then choosing appropriate treatment.

Figure 3.11 illustrates another important point: screw fixation alone provides poor stability against bending and torsional forces (especially

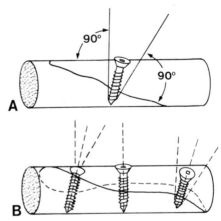

Figure 3.12. Two methods of improving the stability of screw fixation of oblique fractures. A, intermediate angle of screw insertion. B, combined intermediate and perpendicular angles of screw insertion. (Reprinted with permission from M. E. Müller, M. Allgöwer, and H. Willeneger. *Manual of Internal Fixation.* Springer-Verlag, Berlin, 1970.)

bending forces parallel to the axis of the screws). Since most long bones are intermittently subjected to both bending and torsional loads, it is generally recommended that some other form of fixation be used in addition to screws. The *neutralization* plate has been designed to meet this need. The next section "Biomechanics of Plate Fixation" will examine the biomechanics of this device in detail; it is enough to say here that its function is to transmit forces from one area of healthy bone to another, bypassing and protecting an area of fracture.

Figure 3.13 *A* and *B* shows a spinal fracture of the humerus in which a radial nerve palsy developed following closed reduction. The fracture was explored and, because of the long spiral, the surgeon elected to treat it with interfragmental screw fixation alone. Two weeks later the patient rolled over in his sleep and was awakened suddenly by an audible (and painful) snap. The screw fixation had not provided adequate stability

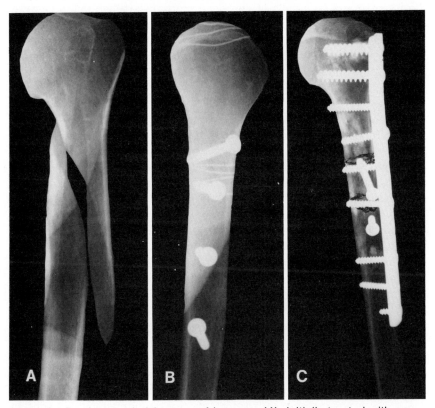

Figure 3.13. Long spiral fracture of humerus (*A*), initially treated with screw fixation alone (*B*). Within 2 weeks refracture occurred. On this occasion, screws and neutralization plate (*C*) had to be used. Fracture healed uneventfully.

against the combined bending and torsional loads and consequently failed. At the second operation a neutralization plate was used in addition to the screw fixation (Fig. 3.13C). This time the fracture healed uneventfully. Though occasionally a long oblique or spinal fracture will heal with screw fixation alone, this should be augmented by a neutralization plate if there is any doubt about the adequacy of the fixation of if it is anticipated that the fracture may be subjected to bending or torsional loads—as in the example cited.

In summary, for any oblique long bone fracture, no single angle of screw insertion provides rigid stability against all load configurations. The optimal angle is determined by the fracture pattern and the predominant load to which the particular bone will be subjected. Adequate stability is achieved in most oblique fractures either by inserting the screw at an angle intermediate between a right angle with the plane of the fracture and the shaft of the bone or by inserting some screws at right angles to the shaft and others at an intermediate angle (Fig. 3.12). If there is any doubt about the stability of the reduction or the types of forces to which the fracture will be subjected, screw and neutralization plate fixation should be combined.

BIOMECHANICS OF PLATE FIXATION

The bone plate has become the most widely used form of internal fixation for long bone fractures. As a result, this device has attracted a great deal of biomechanical interest.[5, 13, 14, 17, 25, 27, 30, 39] Mechanically the plate has two functions: it transmits forces from one end of a bone to the other, bypassing and thus protecting the area of fracture; and it maintains proper alignment of the fragments throughout the healing process.

Contrary to earlier expectations, fracture fixation with plates does not increase the healing rate; in fact, it slows it considerably, and this has been attributed both to periosteal stripping during the operation and the phenomenon of *stress protection.* Stress protection is observed whenever an internal fixation device removes physiological stress from a region of bone and thus removes an important stimulus for healing and remodeling.[12, 15, 34, 35, 37] Diehl and Mittelmeier[15] performed bending tests on human tibiae after removal of steel plates and found the resistance to bending to be diminished by one-third. Torino et al.[33] observed this same reduction in the strength following removal of plates from dog femora. With the development of more rigid forms of internal fixation, stress protection may become a major cause of refracture, following plate removal. A great deal of research is attempting to elucidate this phenomenon and to design implant devices that minimize its effect.[33]

One of the major biological advantages of rigid internal fixation is that it allows early mobilization of the extremity, thereby preventing "cast disease"—muscle atrophy, osteopenia, and other unfavorable effects of immobilization.[27] However, the clinician must always weigh these advantages against the risks of surgery, the knowledge that bone healing may be delayed, and the fact that a second operation will usually be required to remove the device.

Internal fixation of fractures always represents a race between the time required for bone healing and the inevitable fatigue failure of the implant. Although the surgeon has been aided by the development of newer alloys and more rigid fixation devices, his lack of appreciation of the biomechanical principles governing their use continues to be a common cause of failure of internal fixation. The purpose of this section is to explain a number of clinically important principles that apply to plate fixation of long bone.

From a biomechanical viewpoint there are four types of bone plates: neutralization, compression, buttress, and condylar. Each of these has a clearly defined role.

Neutralization Plate

The function of this plate has been alluded to during the discussion of screw fixation. the neutralization plate acts as a "bridge" transmitting forces from one end of the bone to the other, bypassing the area of fracture. Its primary function is to act as a mechanical link between the healthy segments of bone, above and below the fracture, and not to produce interfragmental compression. The most common clinical application of the neutralization plate is to protect screw fixation of short oblique, butterfly and mildly comminuted long bone fractures or in conjunction with bone grafting of a segmental bone defect. Since its major function is to transmit forces from one segment of bone to another, the plate must be rigidly constructed and long enough to ensure good fixation to the proximal and distal fragments. Rules for the proper size and length of neutralization plates have been evolved empirically; however, the Swiss Association for the Study of Internal Fixation (ASIF) has documented and analyzed the data from a large number of patients treated with various forms of internal fixation. This work has produced guidelines in the selection of the proper size and length of neutralization plate for specific long bone fractures. Their text on the techniques and principles of internal fixation is highly recommended.[28]

Compression Plate

There is controversy over whether this should be called a compression or a tension plate. The compression plate produces an axial compression load in the structure to which it is coupled by creating a tension load in the plate (Newton's Third Law: To every action there is always an equal and opposite reaction). By producing axial interfragmental compression, this device can achieve better fracture immobilization than that obtained with a neutralization plate alone.

It has been show experimentally that compression plating produces *rigid* immobilization of fractures and can maintain signficant compression loads for several months after operation.[28, 30] One of the biological characteristics of bone union following rigid immobilization such as that achieved with compression plating is the absence of callous formation around the bone. Bone union occurs by the direct growth of bone from one fragment to the other—called *primary bone union.*[28]

Three techniques are commonly used to carry out a compression plating: tensioning devices, self-compressing plates, and offset screws.

Tensioning Devices

This ingenious device, designed by M. E. Müller,[32] can be coupled between the bone plate and the adjacent bone cortex and then tightened to produce large compression forces across the fracture (Fig. 3.14). Under optimal conditions, this device can create interfragmental compression forces greater than several hundred pounds.[30] The only major disadvantage is that its attachment to the bone requires a larger surgical exposure. In recent years the tensioning device has been supplemented by the self-compressing plate for the treatment of many long bone fractures.

Self-Compressing Plates

A plate utilizing this principle was first described by Bagby[4] in 1956. A number of manufacturers have designed other types of self-compressing

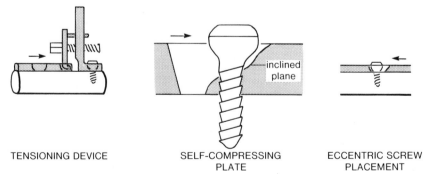

TENSIONING DEVICE | SELF-COMPRESSING PLATE | ECCENTRIC SCREW PLACEMENT

Figure 3.14. Three methods of producing compression plate fixation. (Reprinted with permission from M. E. Müller, M. Allgöwer, and H. Willeneger. *Manual of Internal Fixation.* Springer-Verlag, Berlin, 1970.)

plates based on this principle. In essence, the screw and plate are designed so that as the screw is advanced into the bone, it slides down in an inclined plane that is part of the plate's screw hole (Fig. 3.14). The effect is to create a tension force in the plate and compression forces across the fracture fragments. Under ideal conditions, self-compressing plates are capable of creating compression loads in excess of 200 lb.[30] Thus it is that rigid immobilization of fractures using self-compressing plates has revolutionized the operative management of fractures.

Eccentric Screw Placement

As pointed out earlier ("The Biomechanics of the Screw"), eccentric placement of a screw in a plate hole creates considerable shear stresses in the screw. These same forces are transmitted to the plate and occasionally can be used to produce interfragmental compression. If one wishes to use a standard bone plate (or neutralization plate) to achieve interfragmental compression, the screw can be placed eccentrically in the screw hole (Fig. 3.14). The surgeon should be aware, however, that most bone plates have not been designed for this type of use; consequently, this system is not mechanically efficient and involves the risk that the screws may shear off. It is useful to remember that eccentric screw placement can be used to simulate a self-compressing plate, but the technique has definite limitations.

Buttress Plate

The buttress plate distributes force over a wide area. The mechanical function of this plate is to strengthen (buttress) a weakened area of cortex, and it is most frequently used in treating metaphyseal fractures. By providing cortical stability against compression loading, it prevents the bone from collapsing during the healing process. Because of its buttress function, the plate is usually designed with a large surface area to distribute the loads widely. Common examples of buttress plates are the "T plates" used for tibial plateau (Fig. 3.15) and the Ellis plate for distal radius fractures. Figure 3.16 illustrates how a buttress plate was utilized to "buttress" the weakened medial cortex following open reduction of a severely comminuted tibial plateau fracture.

Condylar Plate

The condylar plate is distinguished from the plates described above, as it carries out a distinct mechanical function. Its main application has been in the treatment of intra-articular distal femoral fractures and its mechanical functions are two-fold (Fig. 3.17A). It maintains the reduction of the major intra-articular fragments, hence restoring the anatomy of

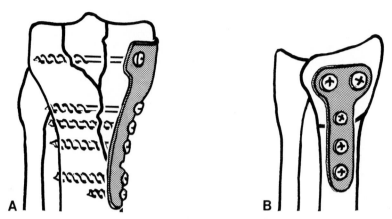

Figure 3.15. Buttress or "T" plates for tibial plateau fractures (*A*) or distal radius fractures (*B*).

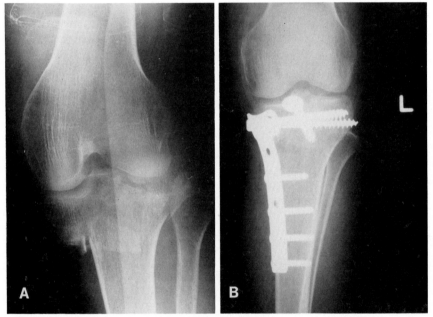

Figure 3.16. Severely comminuted tibial plateau fracture (*A*) treated with elevation of plateau and fixation with lag screw and buttress plate (*B*).

the joint surface, and it rigidly fixes the metaphyseal components to the diaphyseal shaft, permitting early movement of the extremity.

To carry out these two functions requires properties of both the neutralization and buttress plates, and since most of these appliances can be coupled to a tensioning device,[27,28] they also incorporate the advantages of compression plating. Figure 3.17B shows a Y-type intracondylar fracture of the distal femur treated with open reduction and condylar plate fixation. Because of the amount of metaphyseal comminution and fear of loosing axial alignment, we elected not to use the tensioning device for this case. Hence, the buttress plate, like all forms of fixation, must be tailored to the individual fracture.

ADDITIONAL PRINCIPLES OF INTERNAL FIXATION

Several principles concerning the use of the various types of bone plates require elaboration, namely, tension band principle (plate and

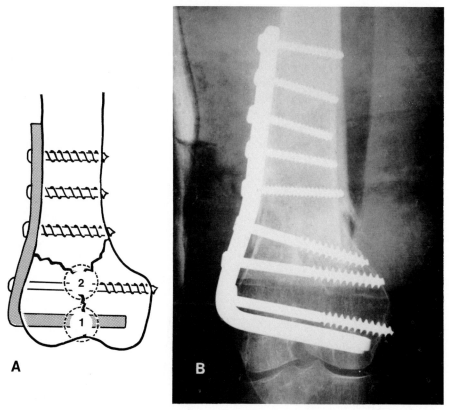

A   B

Figure 3.17.   *A*, the two biomechanical functions of the condylar plate are to maintain the reduction of the major intra-articular fragments (preserving joint congruency) and rigidly fix the metaphysis to the shaft (permitting early joint movement). *B*, example of a condylar plate used for treating a Y-type intracondylar fracture of the distal femur.

wire), concave prebending of plates, plate fixation of oblique long bone fractures, and minimizing the stress concentration at the plate bone junction.

Tension Band Principle

Contrary to popular belief, this expression is not synonymous with compression plating. *Any* device that will resist tension (compression plate, neutralization plate, or steel wire) can be used as a tension band. The common property of all tension bands is that they must be applied to the side of the bone that is normally subjected to tension loads.[28] By placing the fixation device on the tension side of the bone, the surgeon can alter the forces at the fracture line from bending to pure compression, thereby increasing the stability of the fracture.

As Chapter 1 pointed out, it is virtually impossible to apply a purely concentric compression load to a long bone because the bone is not a perfect cylinder and therefore any axially applied load will produce a bending moment (one side of the bone is under compression and the other is under tension). Figure 3.18*A* illustrates how an axially applied load to the femur results in a varus moment, with the lateral cortex under tension and the medial cortex under compression. If the patient had a middiaphyseal fracture, as shown in the figure, with axial loading the lateral cortex would open and the distal fragment would angulate into varus. This unstable fracture can be made stable with a tension band.

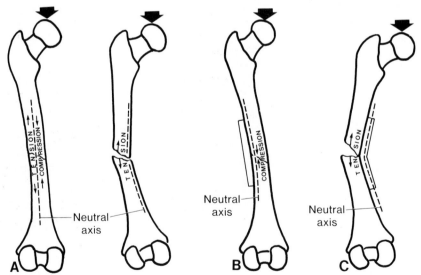

Figure 3.18.   Tension band principle. *A*, no fixation (unstable). *B*, tension band plate (stable). *C*, plate on compression side of bone (less stable).

Figure 3.18*B* illustrates that placing a tension band on the lateral (tension) side of the bone shifts the *neutral axis* from the center of the bone to the junction between the fixation device and the bone. Now, instead of being subjected to both tension and compression loads (i.e., a bending moment), the fracture line is subjected to pure compression, a much more stable situation.

It is important to recall that the tension band will exert its effect whether a compression plate or a neutralization plate is used. The main difference between these two forms of fixation is that the compression plate provides interfragmental compression even when the limb is resting and hence confers an additional degree of stability.

With a tension band in place, any axially applied load will produce tension in the plate and distribute pure compression forces across the fracture (Fig. 3.18*B*). As a result, the stress is dissipated partly by the plate (through tension) and partly through the fracture (through compression, its most stable load configuration).

In contrast, Figure 3.18*C* shows the biomechanical situation that develops when the plate is placed on the *compression* side of the bone. Now the varus bending moment resulting from an axial load tends to open up the fracture, leaving the load to be borne by the plate alone. Obviously this is a much less stable form of fixation than that achieved with a tension band.[6, 22]

When using a tension band plate it is important that the cortices be intact on the side of the bone opposite the plate. If there is any gap or defect in the opposite cortex, the plate will be subjected to bending rather than pure tension loads and will rapidly fatigue and break. Figure 3.19 shows the fixation achieved during the plating of a tibial osteotomy. Note that a wide gap was left between the two cortices opposite the side of the plate. This caused the plate to be subjected to repetitive bending loads, resulting in plate fatigue, and fracture over the ensuing 3 months. A bone plate will only act as a tension band if applied to the tension side of the bone and if there is no bone defect opposite the tension band.[28]

Though the tension band principle is sound, observers in recent years have pointed out that most long bones have NO pure tension or compression side. For example, during gait the lateral cortex of the femur alternates from compression to tension loading, depending on the phase of the gait cycle. As a consequence of this new understanding of long bone mechanics, controversy has arisen concerning which side of a particular long bone represents the "tension" and which represents the "compression" surface. Though this question is still to be fully resolved, for clinical purposes, Table 3.1 lists the commonly recommended sites for placing bone plates to achieve the greatest tension band effect. These

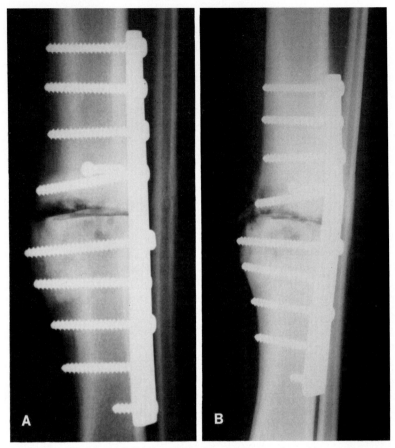

Figure 3.19.   Fixation of tibial osteotomy with bone plate. Note wide gap opposite plate.This produced a bending moment in plate. Over the next 3 months the plate fatigued and fractured (*B*). ALWAYS TRY TO ACHIEVE CORTICAL STABILITY OPPOSITE A COMPRESSION PLATING.

biomechanical considerations, however, have to be modified according to the biological constraints imposed (i.e., availability of skin coverage, etc.) Having decided on which side of the long bone to place the fixation device, the surgeon must then determine whether the plate should be applied as a compression or neutralization plate. This decision usually depends upon the type of fracture configuration. Transverse and short oblique fractures lend themselves best to compression plate fixation because the resulting axial compression load produces mainly interfragmental compression and the shear forces at the fracture line are not excessive (Fig. 3.20). On the other hand, comminuted butterfly and long

Table 3.1 Diaphysial Locations to Optimize Tension Band Principle

Long Bone Diaphysis	Cortex under Maximum Tension
Femur	Anterolateral
Tibia	Variable
Humerus	Posterior
Ulna	Subcutaneous border
Radius	Dorsal

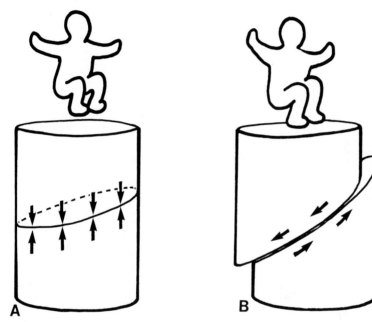

Figure 3.20.   Effect of obliquity of the fracture line on stability. *A*, short oblique fracture primarily has compression forces across the fracture and hence is stable when subjected to axial compression loads. *B*, in contrast, the long oblique fracture has high interfragmental shear forces and hence is more prone to slip under axial loading.

oblique fractures are more commonly treated with neutralization plate fixation, as axial loading in this situation can produce excessive shearing forces at the fracture line, resulting in failure of fixation. However, it is difficult to make generalizations concerning the optimal type of fixation. Each fracture must be judged by its own "personality" (type of bone, type of fracture, location, etc.). This understanding combined with an appreciation of the biomechanics of the various types of fixation devices will guide the surgeon in choosing the optimum mode of treatment.

Tension Band Wiring

Although this is not a form of plate fixation, it is described here as a subsection of the tension band principle. The tension hand wire loop serves the same function as a plate. It converts the forces across the fracture line from bending to pure compression, and hence it adds to the stability of the reduction.

The two commonest examples of tension band wiring are seen in the treatment of transverse fractures of the patella and olecranon. As illustrated by Figure 3.21, there is a close mechanical similarity between these bones; i.e., both bones alter the lever arms about joints, resulting in increased efficiency of the respective extensor muscle groups. As a result, both the patella and the olecranon are subjected to bending forces. By placing a tension band wire on the tension side of these fractures, one ensures that normal muscle activity will place the fracture lines under compression loading. Figure 3.22 illustrates the application of tension band wiring technique in treating fractures of the patella and olecranon.

Concave Prebending of Plates

Fixing a compression plate on the tension side of a long bone counteracts physiological bending forces through the fracture by creating a bending moment in the opposite direction. This moment results from fixing the plate to the outer cortex of the bone, producing an eccentric load. If this principle were carried to its extreme and the compression plate were placed under too much tension, a bending moment could be

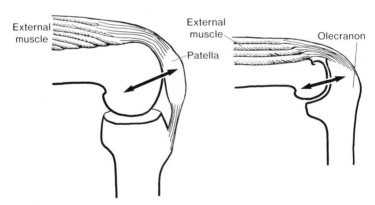

Figure 3.21. Mechanical similarity between patella and olecranon. Both patella and olecranon increase the length of the lever arm, which increases the efficiency of the extensor muscles. Both are subjected to tension and bending loads; the tension side is on the subcutaneous surfaces.

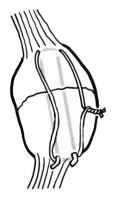 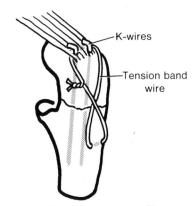

Figure 3.22.   Tension band wiring of patella and olecranon.[28]

produced sufficient to open up the cortex opposite the fracture line[13, 14, 28] (Fig. 3.23).

The technique of *concave prebending* has been developed to compensate for the bending moment produced by the eccentrically applied compression plate load. Here the plate is bent in such a manner that when it is secured to the bone, it produces a compression force along the opposite cortex (Fig. 3.24). By concave prebending, any desired stress pattern across the fracture line can be produced. Ideally, the surgeon should prebend the plate just enough to produce a uniform compression load across the fracture. Diehl[13] has carried out a series of experiments in which he calculated the optimal amount of prebending for each type of bone plate, bone, and amount of interfragmental compression.

Plate Fixation of Oblique Long Bone Fractures

When an oblique fracture is subjected to an axial compression load, shear stresses are produced along the fracture line. The greater the obliquity of the fracture, the higher the shear forces and the greater the tendency of the fragments to slide over on another (Fig. 3.20). To avoid this complication the plate should be applied so as to function as both a *buttress* plate and a *compression* plate. If it is placed over the "tip" of one of oblique fragments and secured firmly to the other fragment before axial compression is applied, the plate will act as a buttress, preventing the sliding of one fragment over the other (Fig. 3.25).

Minimizing Stress Concentration at the Plate Bone Junction

Stress concentration occurs wherever there is a sudden change in the mechanical properties of a structure (Ch. 1). The more abrupt the change, the greater the stress concentration. Since stainless steel is 10 times as

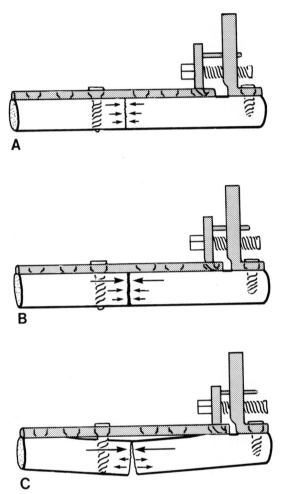

Figure 3.23.   Excessive compression by plate can produce a bending moment and distract the opposite cortex. *A*, mild compression. *B*, moderate compression. *C*, ''over'' compression.

stiff as cortical bone,[29] stress is concentrated at the junction between the end of a plate and the bone. As shown in Figure 3.26, the resulting stress concentration can produce a fracture at this site. To decrease the stress concentration at the end of a bone plate, several investigators have suggested that the screw in the last hole of the plate be inserted into *one* cortex only. Theoretically the *stiffness* of the plate bone complex with a screw in one cortex is lower than that with a screw in both cortices; hence, stress would be concentrated at the plate bone junction more

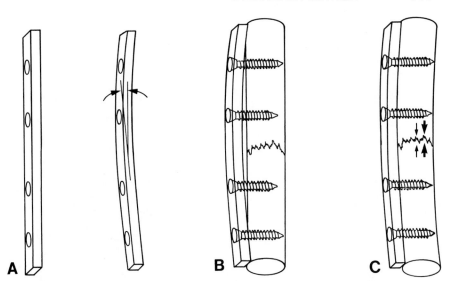

Figure 3.24.   Concave prebending. Plate is "prebent" in a manner (A) such that as it is secured to the bone (B), the cortex opposite the plate is subjected to compression forces (C).

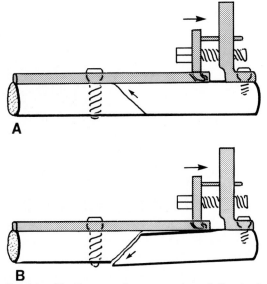

Figure 3.25.   Combined buttress and compression plating techniques for long oblique fractures. By placing compression plate over "tip" of one oblique fragment and securing it firmly to the other fragment before activating tensioning device, the plate will act as a buttress, preventing the sliding of one fragment over the other (A). B shows how fragments override if compression plate is not applied in such a manner as to produce the buttress effect.

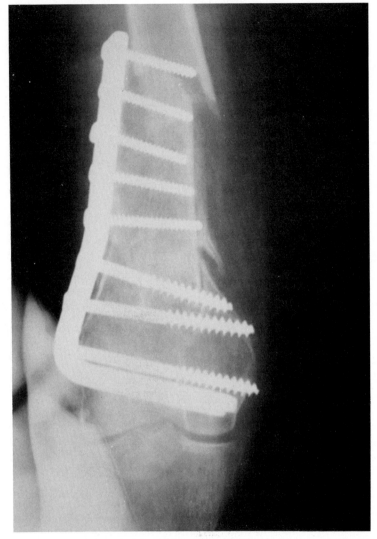

Figure 3.26.   Fracture at junction between plate and bone that occurred 3 months following surgery.

gradually. If the mechanical characteristics are altered less abruptly, the stress concentration is less. Although this theory awaits vigorous experimental proof and is questioned by some, it has already gained considerable clinical popularity. It is described here not to defend its validity but only to explain the rationale behind its use.

BIOMECHANICS OF INTRAMEDULLARY FIXATION

Archeological studies reveal that in ancient times attempts were made to fix long bone fractures using wooden pegs inserted into the medulla. The currently popular form of intramedullary (IM) fixation was said to have been introduced in North America by injured prisoners returning from World War II. The German orthopedist Küntscher[21] developed this technique before the war, and throughout the war it was an accepted form of treatment in Germany. Because it allows almost immediate mobilization of the extremity, IM nailing has rapidly gained popularity during the past two decades. This section will discuss the biomechanics of IM fixation of long bone fractures.

As pointed out earlier, the primary functions of any internal fixation device are to maintain alignment of the fragments during healing and to transmit loads from one end of the bone to the other. Because it is inserted down the center of the shaft and follows the natural contour of the long bone, IM fixation serves these functions well. Although not all long bone fractures are suited for IM fixation, the middiaphysis of the femur is particularly suited for this form of fixation for several reasons:

Shape

The middiaphysis (isthmus) of the femur has a relatively cylindrical medullary canal and is of uniform diameter. This characteristic and its thick, hard cortex make this bone suitable for power reaming and enable it to provide an excellent mechanical link with the IM nail.

Accessibility

The greater trochanter of the femur is an ideal site for the insertion of IM nails. Its superficial location (deep to the ileotibial tract) and the ease with which nails can be inserted through its tip almost make it appear that this bony eminence has been designed for this purpose.

Many surgeons have attempted to develop an easy technique of IM nailing of the tibia. Like the femur, its medullary canal at the isthmus is quite straight and is surrounded by thick cortical bone. Unfortunately, this bone is not easily accessible for IM nail insertion. Lacking a region equivalent to the greater trochanter of the femur, it is necessary to insert the tibial nail near the tuberosity. Unfortunately, the angle of insertion required dictates that either the nail be bent excessively before insertion or that a large window be removed from the cortex, substantially weakening the bone. For this and other reasons, IM fixation of the tibia has never attained the popularity of femoral nailing.

Rotational Tolerance

IM fixation provides excellent axial alignment and good bending resistance but is weakest when subjected to torsional loads. Because the hip and knee can compensate for a mild degree of femoral malrotation or angulatory malalignment, fractures of the femur lend themselves well to IM fixation. In contrast, the forearm bone will not tolerate even a small degree of malrotation because of the intricate relationship between the movements of the ulna and radius during pronation and supination. Hence, IM nailing of forearm fractures has never achieved popular acceptance.

An appreciation of the biomechanics of IM fixations requires an understanding of a number of factors that affect strength of fixation: shape of the nail, diameter of nail, working length, and fixation between nail and bone.

Shape of Nail

Chapter 1 has described how shape confers rigidity to an object. This property is described by the *moment of inertia*. Knowing the stiffness of any material and its moment of inertia, one can calculate its resistance to deformation under various loading conditions. Resistance to bending loads is described by the *area moment of inertia* and resistance to torsional loads by the *polar moment of inertia*.

Biomechanically the ideal IM fixation device would have both high area and polar moments of inertia. However, this design feature must be modified by the practical need for a device that can be easily inserted and will provide good fixation with the bone. Hence, the design of any fixation device represents a compromise.

Stress Strain Curves

The significance of stress-strain curves depends upon an understanding of certain fundamental physical concepts. For example, STRESS IS NOT SYNONYMOUS WITH STRAIN. *Stress* is the internal resistance of a structure to deformation (change of shape), whereas *strain* is the actual change of shape. If a bending or torsional load is applied to an IM nail, stress is produced and a strain results. The stress-strain curve records the amount of strain (deformation) that will result from a given load. From this curve one can determine a number of factors, about the behavior of a structure.

Three currently popular forms of femoral IM fixation are the Schneider, cloverleaf, and diamond-shaped nails. Their biomechanical properties have been compared in an excellent study by Allen et al.[1] Figures 3.27 and 3.28 taken from their work compare the bending and torsional

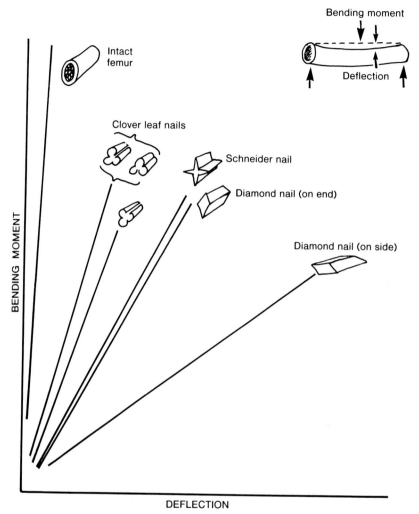

Figure 3.27. Bending characteristic of intact femur compared with that of the cloverleaf nail, Schneider nail, and diamond nail. (Modified and reprinted with permission from W. C. Allen, M. S. Petrowski, A. H. Burstein, et al. Clinical Orthopedics *60:* 13–19, 1968.)

characteristics of the three nails. The actual curves record the strain (horizontal axis) that results from a particular load (vertical axis). For simplicity, the graphs do not provide the actual values of stress and strain, but instead show the relative stiffness of the different nails. The stiffness of each nail is represented by the slope of its curve (also called the modulus of elasticity or Young's modulus). Figure 3.27 compares the bending characteristics of the three types of rods with that of the intact femur, and Figure 3.28 compares the torsional characteristics. From the graphs one can see that each type of nail has certain desirable attributes, but no single nail is optimal for all situations.

Bending Characteristics

Figure 3.27 shows that all three IM nails have less than half the bending stiffness of the intact femur. Of the three rods tested, the cloverleaf nail resists bending most effectively. However, its stiffness depends upon how the nail is loaded; it is most rigid when the slot is located on the tension side. When the slot is placed on the compression side, local "buckling" occurs and the rod fails.[28] For this reason the manufacturers of cloverleaf nails usually recommend that for femoral fractures the nail be inserted with the slot positioned anterolaterally.

The diamond-shaped nail has its greatest bending resistance if it is inserted with its widest diameter (major axis) resisting the load, and, therefore, it should always be inserted in the femur with the major axis facing laterally.

The Schneider nail in its weakest configuration has the same bending rigidity as the diamond nail in its strongest configuration.

Torsional Characteristics

Figure 3.28 compares the torsional characteristics of the three IM rods with those of the intact femur. Again, note that all of the fixation devices are less stiff than the intact bone. The Schneider nail has the most resistance to torsional loads. Its cross-sectional appearance explains its superiority; because its mass is distributed symmetrically around its binding axis, it has the highest *polar moment of inertia*. When subjected to a torsional load, the cloverleaf nail is least rigid because it represents an *open section* (see Ch. 1) and hence has the lowest polar moment of inertia.

The above discussion of bending and torsional characteristics of the IM nail is not intended to show that one type is inherently superior to another, but rather to point out that design differences have evolved for specific reasons. In addition, each type of nail has a recommended method of insertion to maximize its strength characteristics. However, not only does shape affect the strength of an IM nail, but also its diameter, composition, and the degree of fracture comminution (i.e., working length).

Diameter of Nail

There has been a general tendency to use the largest internal fixation device that is practical, especially in the IM fixation of femoral fractures.

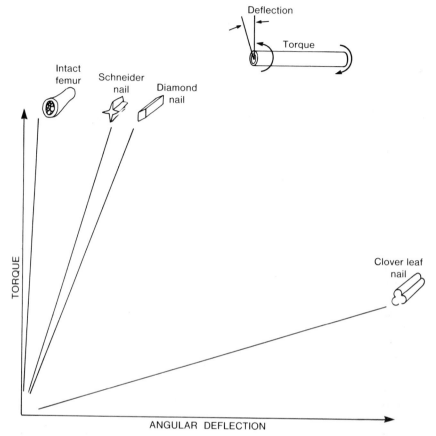

Figure 3.28. Torsional characteristics of intact femur compared with the Schneider nail, diamond nail, and cloverleaf nail. (Modified and reprinted with permission from W. C. Allen, M. S. Petrowski, A. H. Burstein, et al. Clinical Orthopedics *60:* 13–19, 1968.)

One reason for this is that a small increase in the diameter of an IM nail markedly affects its stiffness. For example, a 13-mm cloverleaf nail is less than one and a half times the diameter of a 9-mm nail, and yet its torsional and bending strength is four to five times that of the smaller nail.[1] For the cloverleaf nail, the bending strength is reported to vary with the cube of its diameter; thus, increasing the nail's diameter by 25% doubles its strength.[33] Another reason for the tendency towards large nails is that by reaming the canal and then inserting a large diameter nail, the surgeon is better assured of a good fixation between the nail and the bone. However, the surgeon should appreciate the fact that excessive reaming of the medullary canal can substantially weaken the bone.[11]

Working Length

This concept, which has been described by Allen et al.,[1] has important implications in IM fracture fixation. The working length is the unsupported portion of the nail between the two major bone fragments (Fig. 3.29*C*). Obviously, the greater the working length of the nail the less its resistance to bending or torsional loads. An increase in the working length of a nail has a greater effect on its bending resistance than on its torsional resistance. According to Allen et al.,[1] the bending resistance varies inversely with the square of the working length, while the torsional resistance varies inversely with the working length. Doubling the working length of a nail halves the torsional resistance but reduces the bending resistance by 75%.

Working length becomes important when a surgeon considers IM fixation of a comminuted long bone fracture or of a bone weakened by segmental bone loss. A working length of greater than an inch can seriously compromise the bending rigidity of an IM rod. Figure 3.29*A* shows a femur which has fractured through a metastasis from a breast cancer. As the patient also had multiple visceral metastases, her life expectancy was short. In order to keep her mobile and independent as long as possible, we decided to carry out a Zickle nailing of the fracture (Fig. 3.29*B*). The tumor deposit at the fracture site had produced a large area of segmental bone loss. Though the nail had a good purchase of the proximal and distal fragments of bone, the *working length* appeared to be excessive (Fig. 3.29*C* and *D*). To overcome this defect, the ends of both bones were resected to a level where their structural integrity was ensured, and the segment of unsupported nail between the bone end was encased in a thick shell of methyl methacrylate cement (Fig. 3.29*D*). This use of bone cement increased the rigidity of the IM fixation by decreasing the working length of the nail. As noted above, the fixation was carried out to enable the patient to ambulate early and remain independent up to the time of her death.

Interference Fit

The type of fixation achieved between an IM nail and the bone is called an *interference fit*. This term implies that the nail does not grip the bone uniformly throughout its length but that as it is hammered down the canal, it makes contact with cortical bone irregularities at numerous points. Each of these irregularities provides a point of fixation. The stability of the IM nail depends upon the summation of the numerous fixation points that "interfere" with movement of the nail (interference fit). Obviously the more snug the fit between the nail and the canal, the more stable the fixation, especially against torsional loads.[18, 23, 24] The

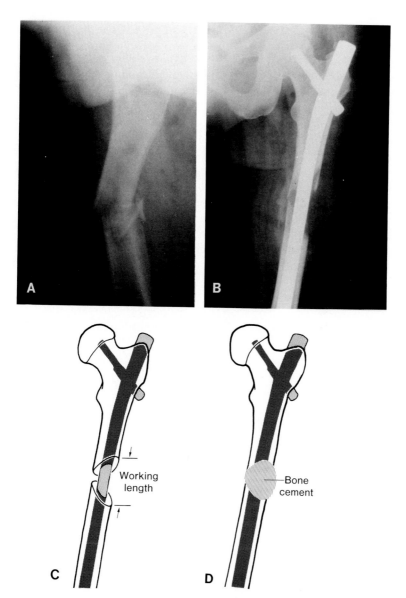

Figure 3.29. *A*, shows a pathological femoral fracture through a metastatic breast cancer. At the time of surgical stabilization with a Zickle nail, it became apparent that the tumor deposit had produced a large segment of bone loss (*B*). Mechanically, the segment of unsupported nail constituted an excessive *working length* (shown diagrammatically in *C*). To overcome this problem, the portion of unsupported nail between the bone ends was encapsulated in a thick shell of methyl methacrylate cement (*D*), reducing the working length of the nail and allowing the patient to remain ambulatory until the time of death from widespread visceral metastasis.

middiaphysis of the femur (isthmus) provides an excellent interference fit because its canal is almost cylindrical and has a uniform diameter. At both ends of the femur the canal "funnels out" rapidly, making firm intramedullary fixation impossible. Because the diameter of the isthmus limits the size of nail that can be inserted, it is difficult to achieve a significant degree of interference fit in regions away from the isthmus.

Küntscher[21] compared the fixation between the IM nail and the diaphyseal cortex to that achieved when a carpenter drives a nail into a block of wood (Fig. 3.30). If the nail is to advance, the wood must be compressed (the solid nail being incompressible). In the case of the cloverleaf nail, the nail *itself* must compress elastically to provide fixation, since the diaphyseal bone is relatively noncompressible after reaming. Küntscher designed the cross-sectional cloverleaf shape to permit compression; the gauge and type of steel are important factors in determining the nail's elasticity.

BIOMECHANICS OF INTERNAL FIXATION

This chapter has elaborated upon a number of important biomechanical principles of screw, plate, and intramedullary fixation as they relate to fracture surgery. The various appliances have been considered in turn.

The screw is a device for converting a torsional load into an axial compression load between the head and the object to which it is applied. The efficiency with which this function is carried out depends upon the use of screws with the optimal design of head, shaft, thread, and tip for each specific application. The orthopedic surgeon should know the advantages and disadvantages of the various designs of orthopedic screw as well as the indications for and contraindications to their use. He should understand the concept of lag fixation and know the optimal angle of screw insertion for various fracture and load configurations.

The bone plate carries out two mechanical functions. It transmits forces from one end of a bone to the other, bypassing and protecting the area of fracture; and it maintains the fracture in proper alignment during the healing process. Although the bone plate allows early mobilization of adjacent soft tissues and joints, this biological advantage must be weighed against the disadvantages of surgical intervention, the consequences of stress protection, and the possibility of fatigue failure of the implant.

There are four types of bone plates: neutralization, compression, buttress, and condylar. Each has a clearly defined role that should be understood by the orthopedic surgeon. The sole function of the *neutralization* plate is to bypass or "neutralize" the forces across a fracture. The *compression* plate achieves axial interfragmental compression by utilizing Newton's third law of physics; this compression can be attained by using

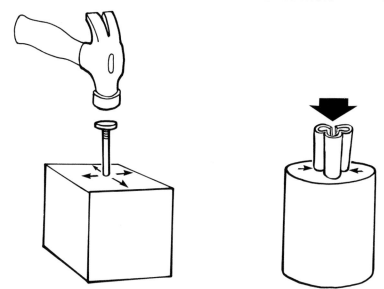

Figure 3.30. Elastic compression. Comparison between the carpenter's nail and the Küntscher cloverleaf nail. The carpenter's nail advances because the wood is compressible, whereas the cloverleaf nail advances because the nail is compressible by virtue of its shape.

a tensioning device or a self-compression plate or through eccentric screw placement in a standard bone plate. The *buttress* plate, used mainly in the treatment of metaphyseal fractures, provides stability against compression loads and prevents the collapse of weakened cortex. The *condylar* plate is used mostly for intra-articular or distal femoral fractures. Its two main mechanical functions are to maintain alignment of the major intra-articular fragments and to securely fix these to the bone shaft. The surgeon should clearly understand which function or combination of functions an internal fixation device is intended to carry out before he uses it.

For proper use of an orthopedic plate, the surgeon should also appreciate the tension band principle, the rationale for concave prebending, and the positioning of a plate to achieve combined compression and buttress plate function in treating oblique long bone fractures.

In applying the biomechanics of IM nailing, the surgeon must understand the concepts of area and polar moment of inertia and how they relate to the mechanical characteristics of a particular design of nail. He should appreciate the limitations of the various types of IM nails commonly used and how each should be inserted to provide maximum structural stability. He should also understand how the strength of a nail is affected by its diameter and "working length" and must be familiar with the concept of interference fit.

This chapter has described a few of the important biomechanical principles that should guide the surgeon in selecting and using the various types of fixation devices available for treating long bone fractures. We have adhered to general principles and have tried to avoid going into detail concerning any one manufacturer's product. It is still the surgeon's responsibility to be thoroughly versed on the specific instructions for any appliance he is about to use. However, he must understand not only the specific instructions regarding a fixation device but also the underlying biomechanical principles governing its correct use.

References

1. ALLEN WC, PETROWSKI MS, BURSTEIN AH, et al: Biomechanics of intramedullary fixation. *Clin Orthop* 60:13–19, 1968.
2. ANSELL RH, SCALES JT: A study of some factors which affect the strength of screws and their insertion and holding power in bone. *J Biomech.* 1:279–302, 1968.
3. ARZIMANOGLOU A, SKIADARISSIS G: Study of internal fixation by screws of oblique fractures in long bones. *J Bone Joint Surg* 34A:219–223, 1952.
4. BAGBY GW: Compression bone plating. *J Bone Joint Surg* 59A:625–631, 1977.
5. BECHTOL CO: Engineering principles applied to orthopedic surgery. *Am Acad Orthop Surg Inst Course Lect* 9:257–664, 1952.
6. BECHTOL CO, MURPHY EF: The clinical applications of engineering principles to the problem of fractures and fracture fixation. *Am Acad Orthop Surg Inst Course Lect* 9:272–275, 1952.
7. BECHTOL CO: The principles of fracture fixation. *Am Acad Orthop Surg Inst Course Lect* 11:92–94, 1954.
8. BECHTOL CO, FERGUSON AB, LAING PG: *Metals and Engineering in Bone and Joint Surgery.* Williams & Wilkins, Baltimore, 1959.
9. BECHTOL CO, LEPPER H: Fundamental studies in the design of metal screws for internal fixation of bone. *J Bone Joint Surg* 38A:1385, 1956.
10. BRITTLE J, HUGHES AN, JORDAN BA: Metallurgical aspects of surgical implant materials. *Injury* 2:225, 1971.
11. CLAUSON DK, SMITH RF, HENSEN ST: Closed intramedullary nailing of the femur. *J Bone Joint Surg* 53A:101–114, 1971.
12. COCHRAN GVB: Effects of internal fixation plates on mechanical deformation of bone. *Surg Forum* 20:469–471, 1969.
13. DIEHL K: Biomechanische Berechnungen und Untersuchungen zur Notwendigkeit der Hohlbiegung bierder Plattenosteosynthese. *Arch Orthop Unfallchir* 80:247–256, 1974.
14. DIEHL K: Festigkeits Berechnungen von Druckplattenosteosynthese im Schaftbereich menschlicher Röhrenknocken. *Arch Orthop Unfallchir* 80:127–141, 1974.
15. DIEHL K, MITTELMEIER H: Biomechanische Untersuchungen zur Erklärung der Spongiosierung bei der Plattenosteosynthese. *Z Orthop* 112:235–243, 1974.
16. FRANKEL VH, BURSTEIN AH: *Orthopedic Biomechanics: The Application of Engineering to the Musculoskeletal System.* Lea & Febiger, Philadelphia, 1970.
17. GOTZEN L, HÜTTER J: Experimentelle Untersuchungen zur plattenvorbiegung—ein Beitrag zur Biomechaik der Plattenosteosynthese. *Arch Orthop Unfallchir* 85:129–138, 1975.

18. HUBBARD MJS: The fixation of experimental femoral shaft torque fractures. *Acta Orthop Scand* 44:55–61, 1973.

19. HUGHES AN, JORDAN BA: The mechanical properties of surgical bone screws and some aspects of insertion practice. *Injury* 4:25–38, 1972.

20. KORANYI E, BOWMAN CE, KNECHT CD, et al: Holding power of orthopedic screws in bone. *Clin. Orthop* 72:283–286, 1970.

21. KÜNTSCHER G: *Practice in Intramedullary Nailing.* Charles C Thomas, Springfield, Ill, 1967.

22. LAURENCE M, FREEMAN MAR, SWANSON SAV: Engineering considerations in the internal fixation of fractures of the tibial shaft. *J Bone Joint Surg* 51B:754–768, 1969.

23. LINDAHL O: Rigidity of immobilization of transverse features. *Acta Orthop Scand* 32: 236–246, 1962.

24. LINDAHL O: Rigidity of immobilization of oblique fractures. *Acta Orthop Scand* 25: 39–50, 1964.

24. LINDAHL O: Rigidity of immobilization with plates. *Acta Orthop Scand* 38:101–114, 1967.

26. LYON WF, COCHRAN JR, SMITH L: Actual holding power of various screws in bone. *Ann Surg* 114:376–384, 1941.

27. MENSCH JS, MARKOLF KL, ROBERTS SB, et al: Experimental stabilization of segmental defects in the human femur. *J Bone Joint Surg* 58A:185–190, 1976.

28. MÜLLER ME, ALLGÖWER M, WILLENEGGER H: *Manual of Internal Fixation.* Springer-Verlag, Berlin, 1970.

29. MURPHY EF: Engineering principles in fracture fixation. *Am Acad Orthorp Surg Inst Course Lect* 11:95–97, 1954.

30. PERRIN SM, MATTER P, RUEDI R, et al: Biomechanics of fracture healing after internal fixation. *Surgery Annual*, 1975, pp 361–390.

31. SCHATZKER J, HOME JG, SUMNER-SMITH G: The effect of movement on the holding power of screws in bone. *Clin Orthop* 111:257, 1975.

32. SMITH H: Surgical technique. In *Campbell's Operative Orthopedics*, edited by AH CRANSHAW. CV Mosby, St. Louis, 1971.

33. SOTO-HALL R, McCLOY NP: Causes and treatment of angulation of femoral intra-medullary nails. *Clin Orthop* 12:66–74, 1953.

34. TORINO AJ, DAVIDSON CL, KLOPPER PJ, et al: Protection from stress in bone and its effects. *J Bone Joint Surg* 58B:107–113, 1976.

35. UHTHOFF HK, DUBRIC FL: Bone structure in the dog under rigid internal fixation. *Clin Orthop* 81:165–170, 1971.

36. UHTHOFF HK: Mechanical factors influencing the holding power of screws in compact bone. *J Bone Joint Surg* 55B:633–639, 1973.

37. UHTHOFF HK: Aktuelle Biomechanische Fragen der Osteosyntheseforchung. *Z Orthop* 113:760–764, 1975.

38. UHTHOFF HK, GERMAIN J: The reversal of tissue differentiation around screws. *Clin Orthop* 123:248–252, 1977.

39. WIRTH CR, CRAWFORD JC, ASKEW MJ, et al: Biomechanics of compression plating. *Surg Forum* 24:470–471, 1973.

Questions—Chapter 3

1. Which of the following screw head designs offers the strongest mechanical coupling between screw and screw driver?
   a. slotted
   b. cruciate
   c. phillips
   d. hexagonal

2. The "pull-out" resistance of a screw is most affected by its:
   a. head design
   b. tip design (self or non-self-tapping)
   c. root diameter of the thread
   d. outside diameter of the thread

3. The breaking strength of a screw is most effected by its:
   a. head design
   b. tip design (self or non-self-tapping)
   c. root diameter of the thread
   d. outside diameter of the thread

4. The most common location of screw breakage is:
   a. midshaft
   b. junction between shaft and thread (Runoff)
   c. midthread
   d. none of above

5. The strength of a screw varies with the —— of its root diameter:
   a. square
   b. cube
   c. fourth power
   d. fifth power

6. For fixation of long oblique fractures, screw insertion perpendicular to the *fracture line* is most effective in resisting the following load configuration:
   a. compression
   b. tension
   c. bending
   d. torsion

7. For fixation of long oblique fractures, screw insertion perpendicular to the *shaft* is most effective in resisting the following load configuration:
   a. compression
   b. tension
   c. bending
   d. torsion

8. The cloverleaf shape intramedullary nail is strongest if inserted so that the slot (open section) is facing the —— side of the bone:
   a. tension
   b. compression

9. The internal forces resisting deformation of a structure are called:
   a. elasticity
   b. stress
   c. strain
   d. plasticity

10. The deformation which occurs in response to an externally applied load is called:
    a. stress
    b. strain

11. Which shape intramedullary nail has the greatest resistance to bending loads?
    a. diamond-shaped
    b. cruciate-shaped (Schneider)
    c. cloverleaf-shaped

12. Increasing the "working length" of a cloverleaf-shaped intramedullary nail has its greatest effect on its resistance to:
    a. torsional loads
    b. bending loads

13. The better the "interference fit" between an intramedullary nail and medullary canal of the bone the greater its resistance to:
    a. torsional load
    b. bending load

14. A transverse middiaphysial long bone fracture is treated with plate fixation. The most rigid fixation will be achieved if the plate is placed on the —— side of the bone:
    a. compression
    b. tension

15. The *polar* moment of inertia describes the —— resistance of a structure:
    a. tension
    b. compression
    c. bending
    d. torsional

16. The *area* moment of inertia describes the —— resistance of a structure:
    a. tension
    b. compression
    c. bending
    d. torsional

17. Which of the following fixation devices best represents an "open section" structure:
    a. bone plate
    b. solid rod
    c. diamond-shaped intramedullary nail
    d. cloverleaf-shaped intramedullary nail

18. Comparing the pull-out resistance of the fluted portion of a self-tapping screw with the fully threaded portion, the fluting decreases the pull-out resistance by:
    a. 10%
    b. 25%
    c. 50%
    d. 80%

19. Which of the following intramedullary devices has the highest polar moment of inertia:
    a. cloverleaf-shaped intramedullary nail
    b. diamond-shaped intramedullary nail
    c. schneider (cruciate shaped) intramedullary nail
    d. triangular-shaped intramedullary nail

20. The bending resistance of a cloverleaf-shaped intramedullary nail increases by the —— power of its outside diameter:
    a. second
    b. third
    c. fourth
    d. fifth

CHAPTER 4

Biomechanics of Pelvic and Acetabular Fractures

Eric R. Gozna

The pelvis performs two major functions: it serves as a protective cage for the abdominal viscera and it provides a mechanical link between the trunk and the lower extremities. Its importance was described by J. B. Howell:[6] "Within its borders are housed a portion of the urinary and intestinal systems and the female genitalia; through its foramina pass the great nerve trunks and blood vessels, while beneath its arches pass all mankind, with few exceptions, the most notable Julius Caesar."

Unlike most other areas of orthopedics, there is remarkably little experimental information on the biomechanics of pelvic and acetabular fractures; the bulk of the information comes from clinical observation alone. One explanation for the lack of experimental data lies in the difficulty of designing such a study. The pelvic ring is remarkably rigid and requires considerable energy to disrupt.[4, 17] Large yet sophisticated testing apparatus is necessary to simulate the complex load configurations involved in pelvic fractures. In addition, it would be a formidable test of the researcher's ingenuity to simulate the dynamic influence of the many muscles that take origin from the pelvis. For these and other reasons there is a paucity of experimental data on the biomechanics of pelvic fractures. However, there is a large body of clinical information, and this chapter will outline some of the more recent concepts concerning the biomechanics of pelvic and acetabular fractures.

As in long bone fracture patterns (Ch. 1), five basic factors determine the manner in which a bone will fracture: two depend upon the characteristics of the bone and three upon the load producing the injury:

Bone characteristics
1. Structural properties of bone
2. Material properties of bone

Load characteristics
1. Type of load
2. Magnitude of load
3. Load rate

Most of our knowledge concerning pelvic mechanics is derived from clinical observation and pertains to the *type of load* and how it relates to the *structural properties* of the pelvis. Little attention has been paid to the influence of *load rate* on fracture patterns. As pointed out in Chapter 1, a viscoelastic material is any material whose mechanical properties depend on the rate at which the load is applied. Bone and most other biological materials are viscoelastic. Also, because of the marked soft tissue "padding" about the pelvis and the varied tissue densities of the abdominal viscera, one would expect this complex to show marked viscoelastic behavior.[4]

The structural properties of the pelvis will be discussed first because this subject provides the key for understanding the biomechanics of pelvic and acetabular fractures; a simple biomechanical model of the pelvis will be developed. The next section will deal with the material properties of the pelvis, and the final section with how load configuration affects the various fracture patterns.

The simple classification of acetabular and pelvic fractures presented here is based upon the concept of force vectors and shows how they relate to the simple biomechanical model of the pelvis.

STRUCTURAL PROPERTIES OF THE PELVIS

It is remarkable that a structure like the pelvis, which is composed mainly of cancellous bone with a thin cortex, should have such enormous strength. The structural properties of the pelvis exemplify how shape influences rigidity. To fully appreciate this relationship, one must study the bony architecture of the pelvis and examine its ligamentous, tendinous, and soft tissue supports (vide infra).

Understanding the bony architecture is difficult if one visualizes the pelvis only in terms of the routine anteroposterior (AP) and lateral pelvic x-rays, because the pelvis and acetabuli slope at angles of approximately 40 to 45° with the horizontal. Special x-ray projections must be used to provide adequate data for a full radiological interpretation of pelvic structures.

Pelvic Views

As will be seen later, the pelvic ring is the main structural unit of the pelvis. To understand the pathomechanics of major pelvic fractures, radiographs should be obtained that delineate clearly the pelvic ring. The ring is best illustrated using the *inlet* and *tangential* pelvic views described by Pennal and Sutherland.[12] Figure 4.1 shows how the x-ray camera should be positioned to obtain these views, with the corresponding diagrammatic representations of the ring and pelvis. The x-ray beam is

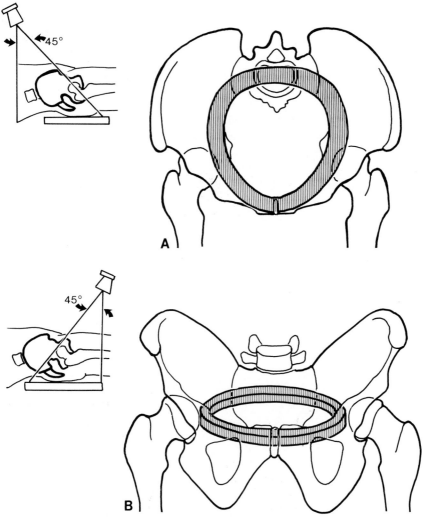

Figure 4.1.   Inlet and tangential views of pelvis are obtained by directing the x-ray camera perpendicular and tangential to the pelvic ring. These views allow the surgeon to determine the exact degree of displacement for any pelvic ring fracture.[12]

angled to produce orthogonal projections of the pelvic ring, one perpendicular and the other tangential to the ring. Because the ring slopes approximately 45° with the horizontal, these two views are obtained by directing the x-ray beams 45° caudad and 45° cephalad. The Pennal pelvic views have greatly aided our understanding of pelvic ring fractures.

Acetabular Views

The acetabuli and their supporting structures are best shown by the "three-quarter oblique" acetabular views described by Judet and Judet.[7] These investigators have won general support for the concept that the acetabuli are supported in the concavity of an arch formed by two columns of bone, the anterior and posterior columns. Anatomically, the *anterior column* corresponds to the iliopubic arch and the superior pubic ramus, while the *posterior column* corresponds to the ileoischial arch (Fig. 4.2). Because the acetabuli slope at an angle of 45° with the horizontal, their margins and the anterior and posterior columns are best delineated using the Judets' three-quarter oblique views (Fig. 4.3). The *internal oblique view* shows the anterior column and the posterior lip of the acetabulum while the *external oblique view* shows the posterior column and the anterior lip of the acetabulum. Since the AP projection

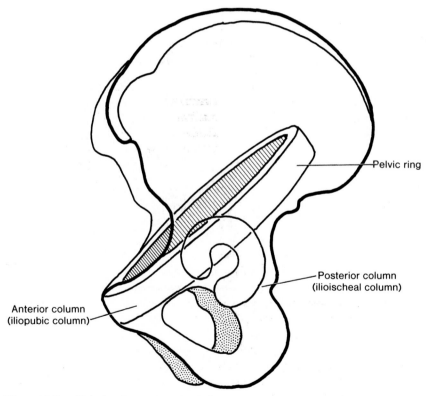

Pelvic ring

Posterior column
(ilioischeal column)

Anterior column
(iliopubic column)

Figure 4.2.   Relation between acetabulum, pelvis ring, and anterior and posterior columns. Note that the anterior column corresponds to the anterior portion of pelvis ring.[7]

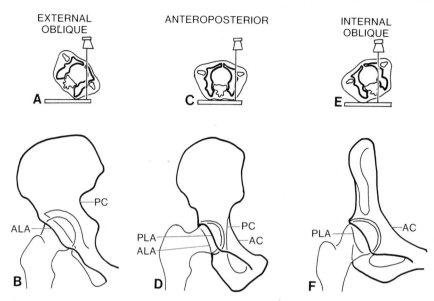

Figure 4.3.   Judet's oblique views of acetabulum.[7] *A* and *E* show how the patient is positioned for oblique views. *External oblique* projection (*B*) outlines the posterior column (*PC*) and the anterior lip of the acetabulum (*ALA*). *Internal oblique* projection (*F*) outlines the anterior column (*AC*) and the posterior lip of the acetabulum (*PLA*). The routine *anteroposterior projection* (*C* and *D*) superimposes the two columns and the two acetabular margins, making x-ray interpretation of fracture patterns difficult. (Reprinted with permission from R. Judet and J. Judet. *Journal of Bone and Joint Surgery* 46A: 1615–1646, 1964.)

shows the columns and the acetabular margins superimposed one upon the other, it is difficult to analyze acetabular fracture patterns from this view alone.

The surgeon must appreciate fully the radiographic anatomy of the pelvis if he is to understand the biomechanics of pelvic and acetabular fractures. The Pennal and Judet views will greatly aid him. Note from Figure 4.3 that the anterior column (iliopubic ramus) in the Judet views corresponds to the anterior portion of the pelvic ring in the Pennal views.

Biomechanical Model

Though from routine radiographs the structure of the pelvis appears complex, biomechanically it can be reduced to several simple components. Biomechanically the pelvis combines the structural attributes of the ring, the column, and the triangle. Figure 4.4 shows how the pelvic structure can be reduced to these simple mechanical components and, for comparison, Figure 4.5 shows the mechanical model as it would appear in the

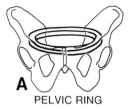

A

PELVIC RING

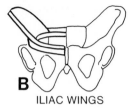

B

ILIAC WINGS

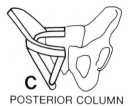

C

POSTERIOR COLUMN

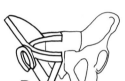

D

ACETABULUM

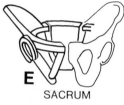

E

SACRUM

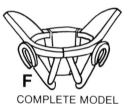

F

COMPLETE MODEL

Figure 4.4.   Diagram illustrating the development of a simple biomechanical model of the pelvis. Model begins with the pelvic ring (*A*), to which is added the iliac wings (*B*), followed by the posterior column and inferior pubic ramus (*C*). The acetabulum is positioned at the apex of the triangle formed by anterior and posterior columns (*D*). The sacrum can be represented by a wedge-shaped structure in the posterior ring (*E*). The complete biomechanical model of the pelvis consists of a ring with two dependent equilateral triangles, the apex of which provides a firm support for the acetabuli (*F*).

standard AP projection, the Pennal pelvic views and the Judets oblique views. Figures 4.5 and 4.6 are comparable projections of the pelvis and acetabuli and illustrate how the model aids in understanding the complex structure of the pelvis. The components of the model can now be described individually.

Pelvic Ring and Anterior Column

The pelvic ring is the single most important structural component of the pelvis. Not only does the ring form most of the pelvic mass, but all of the other components of the pelvis—the posterior columns, acetabular rings, and iliac crests—radiate symmetrically from its periphery.

Anatomically the inner margin of the pelvic ring consists of the body, ala of the sacrum and sacroiliac joints posteriorly, the arcuate lines of the ilia laterally, and the superior pubic rami and symphysis pubis anteriorly (Fig. 4.1).

In the erect position the weight of the body is transmitted down the spine, across the sacroiliac joint, on through the post column and dome

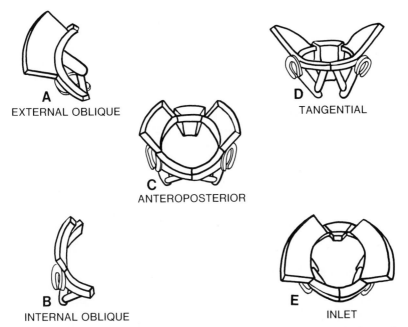

A EXTERNAL OBLIQUE

C ANTEROPOSTERIOR

D TANGENTIAL

B INTERNAL OBLIQUE

E INLET

Figure 4.5.   Biomechanical model as it would appear in anteroposterior projection (*C*), Judet's oblique acetabular views (*A* and *B*), and Pennal's pelvic views (*D* and *E*).

of the acetabulum and on to the head of the femur. This portion of the pelvis contains most of its mass and, because of its important weight-bearing function, is referred to as the "femoral-sacral arch."[1, 3, 4, 11] The trapezoidal-shaped sacrum fits into the pelvic ring much like the keystone of a Roman arch, adding to the structural rigidity of the femoral-sacral arch.[2] Several investigators[3, 4, 11] have pointed out that whereas the posterior portion of the pelvic ring is under compression loading when man is in the erect posture, the anterior portion of the ring is loaded under tension; hence, the anterior ring acts as a "tie beam" to the femoral-sacral arch. These biomechanical facts help explain why the anterior portion of the pelvic ring is so much lighter and has a smaller cross-sectional area than does the posterior position; that is, it is not subjected to the same magnitude of compression loading.

The major supporting structure of the anterior aspect of the pelvic ring is the superior pubic rami and its extension on to the ischium. This area, which Judet and Judet[7] referred to as the *anterior column*, plays an important role in acetabular fractures (see below).

Although the traditional distinction between "stable" and "unstable"

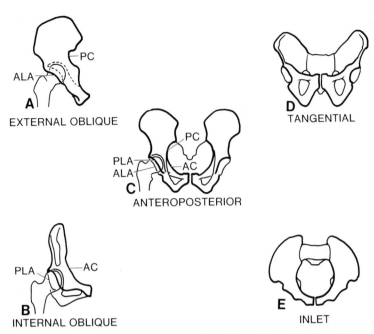

Figure 4.6. Diagrammatic x-ray views of pelvis and acetabuli as they would appear in standard anteroposterior projection (*C*), Pennal's tangential and inlet projections (*D* and *E*), and Judet's oblique acetabular views (*A* and *B*). These views can be compared with similar projection for the biomechanical model in Figure 4.5. *PC*, posterior column; *AC*, anterior column; *PLA*, posterior lip of acetabulum; *ALA*, anterior lip of acetabulum.

pelvic fractures has been based upon the integrity of the pelvic ring,[1, 9, 12] recent findings have challenged this simplistic approach. For example, Gertzbein and Chenoweth[5] have shown with radioisotope techniques that even isolated rami fractures, so common in geriatric patients, are frequently associated with significant injury to the pelvic ring complex. In contrast, Sullivan[17] has pointed out that patients can return to heavy manual labor even after excision of the anterior portion of the pelvic ring. Hence, orthopedic surgeons have come to think of all fractures in terms of a "spectrum of stability" and to assess each fracture in terms of its individual merits.

Iliac Wings

These come off the pelvic ring superolaterally and flare out like fan-shaped plates on each side of the pelvis (Fig. 4.4). As well as protecting the abdominal viscera, the iliac wings provide a strong laterally placed prominence from which the supporting muscles of the lower extremity and trunk originate. They provide stability, like the cross arms on the mast of a sailing ship; hence the ilium is an important mechanical link between the axial skeleton and the lower extremities. Most fractures involving the iliac crests are due to avulsion (tension) loads or a direct blow (compression) to the rim of the crest.

Posterior Column

This term, which was popularized by Judet and Judet,[7] refers to the thickened portion of ischium that runs slightly medially and anteroinferiorly at an angle of 60° from the pelvic ring (Fig. 4.7). The anterior

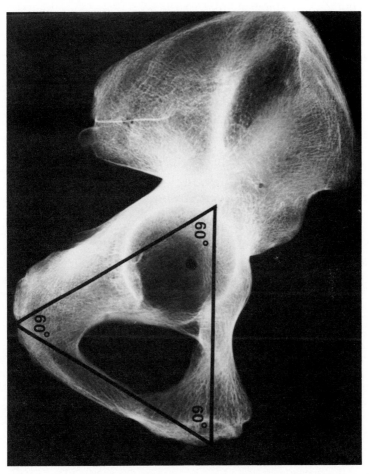

Figure 4.7. X-ray of a disarticulated pelvis, showing how the anterior column (iliopubic column), posterior column (ilioischeal column), and inferior pubic ramus form an equilateral triangle, with a 60° angle between each side. Note how the acetabulum rests in the arch formed by the anterior and posterior columns.

column (superior pubic ramus plus the arcuate line), the posterior column (posterior border of the ischium), and the inferior pubic ramus form a rigid equilateral triangle which supports the acetabulum in its thickened superior apex.

Inferior Pubic Rami

Though its cross-sectional area is small compared with the other structures of the pelvis, the inferior pubic ramus completes the important triangular support of the acetabulum (Fig. 4.7). The inferior pubic rami also provide important ligamentous and tendinous attachments and are important as a mechanical link with the legs.

Acetabulum

This structure, which can be represented as an inverted "U" or horseshoe, is formed from the fusion of three epiphyseal centers which constitute the dome and the posterior and anterior walls of the acetabulum. The dome is the most massive portion, as the major weight-bearing forces are transmitted through this area.[2, 11, 14] Some investigators feel that an important prognostic factor influencing the outcome of central fracture dislocations is the surgeon's ability to keep the femoral head (reduced) beneath an intact acetabular dome.[8, 14] Hence the dome plays an important role in acetabular fractures.

Structurally the massive dome of the acetabulum is well designed to accommodate axial loading in the erect position; however, the absence of any supporting structure inferiorly (i.e., the presence of the acetabular notch) weakens the anterior and posterior lips of the acetabulum. This explains in part why less energy is required to produce anterior and posterior lip fractures than dome fractures. Mechanically the acetabulum would be less prone to these fractures if it had evolved as a complete circle rather than an inverted U.

Sacrum and Sacroiliac Joint

Dommisse[3] emphasized the importance of this part of the femoral-sacral arch. It affords stability by virtue of three factors: the complex concavoconvex shape of the sacroiliac joint surface, which provides stability in a number of planes; the small but effective "shelf" which is formed anteriorly by the iliac component of the sacroiliac joint; and the strong posterior and interosseous ligaments. A great deal of research remains to be done on the biomechanics of the sacroiliac joints.

Ligamentous Supports

Because the bony pelvis is massive and the overlying soft tissue is abundant, little attention has been paid to the contribution of ligaments to pelvic stability. To understand the biomechanics of pelvic fractures, the surgeon should have a keen appreciation of its ligamentous supports. The most extensive ligamentous complexes surround the sacroiliac joints and symphysis pubis. The posterior sacroiliac ligament is the major ligamentous structure stabilizing the posterior pelvic ring, and the anterior interpelvic ligaments provide the major ligamentous support for the symphysis pubis. As would be expected from biomechanical principles, the most rigid ligamentous supports are situated farthest from the center of the pelvic ring, where they have their greatest mechanical advantages. An understanding of the ligamentous supports of the pelvis is essential when planning the treatment of pelvic fractures.

MATERIAL PROPERTIES OF THE PELVIS

A considerable body of data suggests that cancellous bone has important shock-absorbing properties,[4] a fact that explains the predominance of cancellous bone in the region of joints. Since its material characteristics are intermediate between those of soft cartilage and stiff cortical bone, cancellous bone represents a transitional structure which reduces the stress concentration. The greater the forces across a joint, the greater the mass of cancellous bone required to carry out this shock-absorbing function.

The pelvis is composed mainly of cancellous bone because it contains five major joints, all within a radius of less than 3 inches. Though a good shock absorber, cancellous bone is a weaker material than cortical bone; hence, for strength the pelvis must rely heavily on its bulk and structural configuration.

TYPE OF LOAD

Most of the investigation into pelvic fracture mechanics has been directed to determining how the type of load and its line of application affect the fracture pattern. The reader will recall that most of this information is based on clinical observation and not on rigid experimental data. However, these observations have stood the test of time and illustrate several important biomechanical principles. In the following discussion, pelvic and acetabular fractures will be considered under separate headings.

As noted in Chapter 1, the four major load configurations which produce fractures are tension, compression, bending, and torsion. Because of the considerable movement permitted through the hips and spine, it is difficult to apply effective bending and torsional forces to the pelvis. Consequently, the two common load configurations producing pelvic damage are compression and tension. In general, the *tension* (traction) loads result in simple avulsion fractures, while *compression* loads produce significant pelvic and acetabular disruptions.[17]

To appreciate the mechanisms of pelvic and acetabular fractures, it is helpful to understand the concept of a *force vector*. A vector is any quantity that has a magnitude, direction, and point of application.

Magnitude

Most pelvic fractures are the result of high energy loads,[4, 18] especially those injuries that produce instability of the pelvic ring or disruption of major supporting structures, such as the posterior column. Because of the high energy loads necessary to produce major pelvic fractures, the clinician dealing with these injuries should always consider the possibility of associated visceral injuries. Seventy percent of severe pelvic fractures are the result of motor vehicle accidents;[15] many of the patients have associated visceral injuries,[1] and the mortality rate still approaches 10%.[17]

Because the associated injuries usually take precedence over the pelvic fractures, they are often neglected during the initial treatment phase. Often, when the life-threatening situation has been dealt with and the soft tissue injuries have healed, the patient is left to cope with a neglected pelvic fracture.

For acetabular fractures, the most obvious indicator of the magnitude of the force vector is the degree of comminution and the amount of bone disruption. Obviously, higher energy forces are required to produce major acetabular dome disruption than are required to break off a small chip of the posterior acetabular lip.

It is generally not appreciated that compression forces are not equally distributed over the surface of the hip joint but assume a parabolic distribution (Fig. 4.8) because of the compressible nature of articular cartilage and the spherical shape of the joint.[7] The forces would not be so distributed if the articular surface were not compressible; conversely, the more compressible the articular cartilage the higher the stress concentration.

Direction

Pennal[5] and Sutherland[12] has demonstrated that the major force vectors in *pelvic* fractures are distributed along three basic planes—anteroposterior, lateral, and vertical—and for this reason most pelvic fracture patterns can be classified according to these primary vector directions.

For *acetabular* fractures, the direction of the force vectors often can only be summarized retrospectively from the radiological fracture pattern because no one knows the position of the hip at the time of impact. However, the point of maximum articular damage to the femoral head

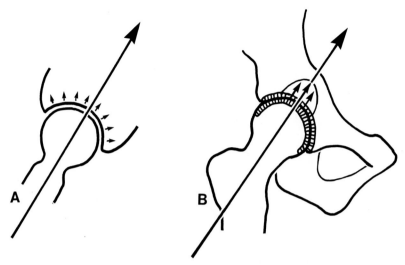

Figure 4.8.   Stress distribution across the hip joint. If the hip were a true ball and socket joint (*A*) with perfect surface congruity and a noncompressible joint surface, stress concentration with weightbearing would be evenly distributed across its surface. In the actual situation (*B*), the noncongruous and compressible articular surface results in an uneven stress distribution. Maximum stress concentration occurs along the line of the force vector and falls off towards the periphery. (Reprinted with permission from R. Judet and J. Judet. *Journal of Bone and Joint Surgery* 46A: 1615–1646, 1964.)

can be determined if the surgeon knows where the force was applied to the leg (by the presence of hematoma, abrasion, or other evidence of local trauma). Because the hip is a ball-and-socket joint, all force vectors must pass through the center of the femoral head (center of rotation). By drawing a straight line on the radiograph joining the point of application of the load with the center of the femoral head, the direction of the force vector can be defined. The point of maximum femoral articular damage should fall along this line (Fig. 4.9).

Point of Application

As will be demonstrated, the point of load application is most important in determining the various *pelvic* fracture configurations; for example, an anterior blow to the symphysis pubis will produce a "straddle" fracture pattern while a blow centered over the anterior iliac crest will produce an "open book" pattern.

In *acetabular* fractures, the point of application of the force vector corresponds to the area of maximum acetabular damage, e.g., centrally, superiorly, posteriorly, etc. This area can usually be determined radio-

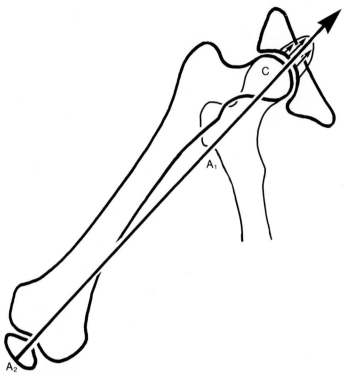

Figure 4.9. The acetabular stress distribution resulting from a blow to the greater trochanter with the hip in neutral position (A_1) is the same as would result from a blow to the anterior aspect of the knee (A_2) with the hip abducted 45°. Hence, the clinician should always examine the knee in any acetabular fracture or hip dislocation. Conversely, one should always obtain x-rays of the hip in any femoral shaft fracture. *Note:* the load vector always passes through the center of the femoral head *(C)*. (Reprinted with permission from R. Judet and J. Judet. *Journal of Bone and Joint Surgery* 46A: 1615–1646, 1964.)

graphically, or else it can be determined if one knows the point on the extremity where the load was applied, e.g., knee, greater trochanter, etc., and the position of the extremity at the time of impact. This information permits one to draw the force vector on the radiograph and determine the point where the vector passes across the acetabulum (areas of maximum damage).

Judet and Judet[7] (Fig. 4.9) pointed out that the acetabular force resulting from a blow to the greater trochanter and directed up the neck of the femur is the same as would occur if the force were applied to the knee with the hip abducted to 45°. This observation has considerable clinical significance in view of the frequent coexistence of knee injuries

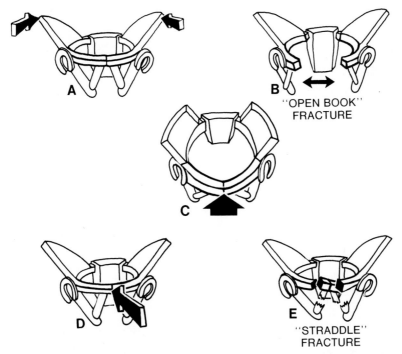

Figure 4.10. Acetabular fracture patterns resulting from a force vector along the course of the femur, with the hip in various positions of flexion and abduction. (Reprinted with permission from R. Judet and J. Judet *Journal of Bone and Joint Surgery* 46A: 1615–1646, 1964.)

and fracture dislocations of the hip.[18] The same pattern of acetabular fracture can result from a blow to the greater trochanter or to the knee, with the hip abducted. In the former situation the surgeon needs to deal with the acetabular fracture alone, but in the latter case he should look for an occult associated knee injury. Hence, the surgeon who thinks in terms of force vectors and attempts to determine where the load was applied to the extremity will be much less likely to miss a significant knee injury associated with an acetabular fracture.

Figure 4.10 shows the types of acetabular fracture patterns that can be anticipated from axially applied loads, with the femur in various positions of flexion and abduction.

Pelvic Fractures

Our understanding of the pathomechanics of pelvic fractures has been greatly advanced by the work of Pennal. Assisted by the radiological expertise of Sutherland and the engineering studies of Garsythe, he

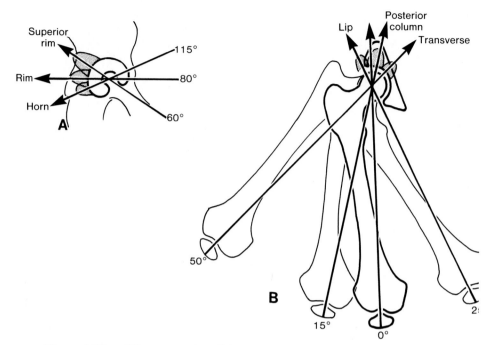

Figure 4.11. AP compression. If force vector is applied centrally, "straddle" pattern (*A*) occurs; if applied laterally, "open book" pattern (*B*) occurs.

devised a practical classification of major pelvic ring fractures based on radiological appearance and correlated this with the direction of load.[12] The three basic fracture patterns described in their classification are the result of three load configurations: anteroposterior compression, lateral compression, and vertical shear. This classification is similar to the one described by Pick[13] in 1955.

Anteroposterior Compression

Two basic fracture patterns can result from a compression load applied across the pelvic ring in an AP direction (Fig. 4.11). Either the four pubic rami fracture off, producing the "straddle"[10] fracture, or the pelvic ring separates anteriorly through the area of the symphysis and opens up like a book (occasionally this is called an "open book" or "hinge" fracture). The *straddle* pattern commonly results from a direct blow to the anterior midline of the ring (symphysis pubis), while the *open book* pattern results from a more laterally placed blow, such as one applied to the anterior aspect of the knee, with the hip flexed to 90°.[3, 12]

An appreciation of the mechanism of injury and the anatomy of the pelvis permits the surgeon to plan a rational treatment protocol. Because of the proximity of both these fractures to the urogenital diaphragm, there is a high incidence of associated injury to the bladder-urethra complex. In the open book injury, the strong posterior sacroiliac ligaments are intact and the book can be closed again, since the bookbinding is still intact. This is usually accomplished by nursing the patient in the supine or lateral recumbent position.[12] If this treatment does not reduce the fracture spontaneously, the surgeon can do a closed reduction or maintain the patient in a hip spica or pelvic sling. Figure 4.12 shows the radiological appearance of a "straddle" pelvic fracture pattern that resulted from a motor vehicle accident in which the patient sustained a direct blow to the symphysis. Fortunately no bladder or urethral injury occurred.

Lateral Compression

Two fracture patterns result from this load configuration: the ipsilateral compression fracture and the contralateral or "bucket handle" fracture (Fig. 4.13).

In the *ipsilateral compression* fracture as described by Pennal and Sutherland[7] the ipsilateral posterior sacroiliac joint is disrupted and the ipsilateral pubic is fractured. In this injury a spike of bone from the rami frequently punctures the bladder wall and, because of the posterior

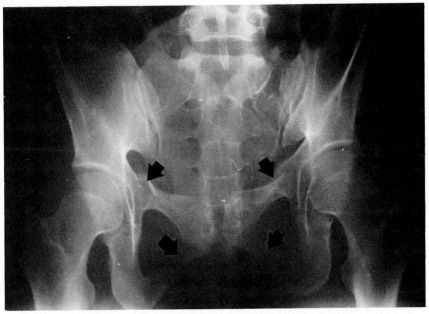

Figure 4.12. X-ray of AP compression "straddle" fracture pattern.

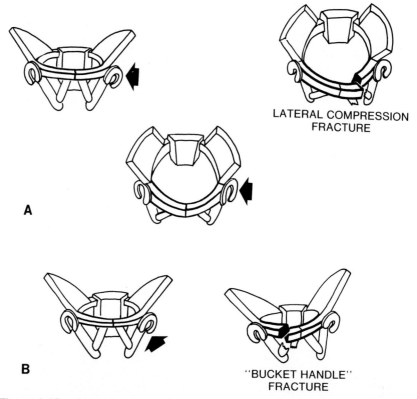

LATERAL COMPRESSION FRACTURE

"BUCKET HANDLE" FRACTURE

Figure 4.13.   Lateral compression. If force vector is applied laterally, ipsilateral fracture pattern (*A*) occurs; if applied from inferolateral direction, hemipelvis rotates, producing either "bucket handle" or contralateral compression patterns (*B*).

sacroiliac disruption, the lumbosacral roots are commonly stretched or avulsed. Frequently this fracture can be reduced by applying external rotation force through the femur, and reduction can be maintained with a hip spica.

The *contralateral or bucket handle* fracture differs slightly from the pure lateral compression fracture in that the force vector is applied from an inferolateral direction instead of a straight lateral direction. Though the predominant force is still one of compression, a rotational moment is also present. As a result, the ipsilateral hemipelvis is rotated upwards, producing the characteristic bucket handle appearance. Reduction of this fracture requires both external rotation and traction through the ipsilateral femur. Pennal and Sutherland[12] and Pick[13] have pointed out that this injury frequently produces disruption of the *contralateral* pubic rami and the ipsilateral sacroiliac region. Hence, the bladder is not as prone to puncture as in the ipsilateral compression fracture (Fig. 4.14).

Vertical Shear

This pattern results from a vertically directed force applied to the inferior aspect of one hemipelvis (Fig. 4.15), as from a fall, landing on the ischial tuberosity or, more commonly, from an axial force along the extended and slightly abducted femur.[12] The involved hemipelvis is separated from the other hemipelvis and trunk, and is completely unstable. Associated injuries to the abdominal viscera and lumbosacral plexus (especially the L5 component) are common. Unfortunately, this is the commonest major pelvic ring fracture pattern. Because of the marked instability of this fracture, maintenance of a reduction is difficult and often requires a long period of immobilization in traction or else surgical stabilization.[12]

Acetabular Fracture Patterns

Anyone interested in the pathomechanics of acetabular fractures should read the excellent work of Judet and Judet.[7] They devised a useful

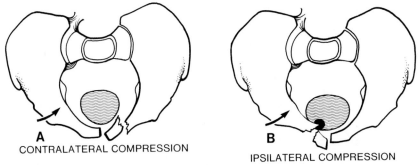

A CONTRALATERAL COMPRESSION

B IPSILATERAL COMPRESSION

Figure 4.14. *A*, contralateral compression fracture—has less tendency to rupture bladder. *B*, ipsilateral compression fracture—frequently associated with disruptions of the posterior sacroiliac ligament complex and bladder injury.

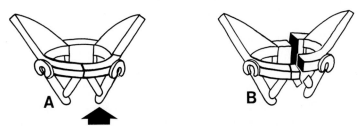

Figure 4.15. Vertical shear. AP vertical or cephalad force vector (*A*) shears off hemipelvis, producing vertical shear pattern (*B*).

classification of these fractures based on careful clinical observation and established several important principles concerning acetabular fracture biomechanics. In the 173 cases studied, almost 70% of the fractures belonged to one of four simple patterns. These patterns and their relative incidence are:

Transverse fracture	43%
Posterior rim fracture	33%
Isolated anterior column fracture	10%
Isolated posterior column fracture	5%

Transverse Fracture

This, the most common fracture pattern, usually results from a blow to the lateral aspect of the great trochanter. The resultant force vector is directed along the neck, through the center of the head and into the central portion of the acetabulum. The fracture line runs transversely across the acetabulum, dividing the innominate into a superior and an inferior portion (Fig. 4.16). As would be expected from biomechanical principles (Ch. 1), the fracture line passes through the region with the lowest *section modulus*, i.e., from the anterior inferior iliac spine, across the acetabular fossa, and out through the sciatic notch.

In the "T" fracture, an uncommon variant (<2%) of the transverse pattern, a secondary fracture line extends inferiorly through the acetabular notch and across the inferior pubic rami (Fig. 4.17).

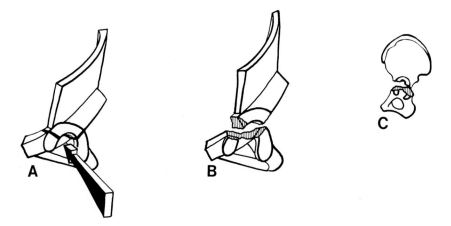

Figure 4.16.   Transverse acetabular fracture. Force vector directed into central portion of acetabulum (*A*) produces transverse fracture (*B*), dividing innominate through acetabulum (*C*).

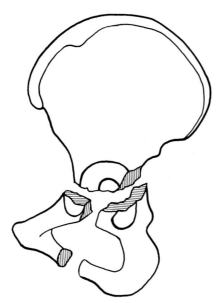

Figure 4.17. "T" fracture is a variation of the transverse pattern in which secondary fracture line is produced inferiorly through acetabular notch.

Posterior Rim Fracture

Fractures of the posterior acetabular lip with dislocation of the femoral head are common in motor vehicle accidents. Frequently the seated occupant (hip flexed and slightly adducted) is thrown forward, striking the knee against the dashboard. The posteriorly directed force vector breaks off the rim of the acetabulum and the hip dislocates. Because of the proximity of the sciatic nerve, palsies are frequent.[16] Depending on the direction and magnitude of the force vector, the acetabular and posterior columns suffer varying degrees of damage. The more hip abduction, the greater the size of the posterior lip fragment and the greater the energy level required to produce the fracture.

Figure 4.18 illustrates the biomechanics of this injury.

Anterior Column Fracture

Isolated fractures of the anterior column are uncommon. These fractures, which result from an anterosuperiorly directed force vector, cause a separation of the anterior column from the rest of the innominate (Fig. 4.19). The fracture line passes through the segment of bone that is structurally weakest (low section modulus); this segment runs from the psoas groove or just above the anterior inferior iliac spine, across the

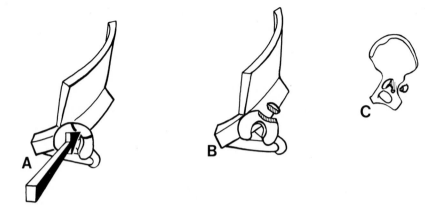

Figure 4.18.   Posterior rim fracture. Posteriorally directed force vector (*A*) shears off rim of acetabulum (*B* and *C*). Portion of rim destroyed depends on position of femur at time of impact (Fig. 4.10).

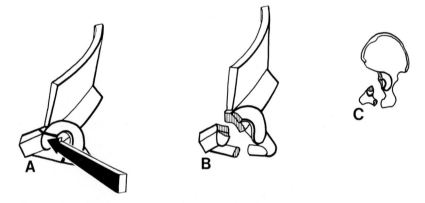

Figure 4.19.   Anterior column fracture. Anteriorly directed force vector (*A*) separates anterior column from rest of innominate (*B* and *C*).

acetabulum into the notch, down into the obturator foramen, and across the inferior pubic ramus. On the radiograph this fracture may be easily confused with the transverse pattern if the oblique views are not carefully studied (these views show the posterior column to be intact).

Judet and Judet[7] believe that this fracture is most frequent following a blow to the greater trochanter with the hip externally rotated.

Isolated Posterior Column Fracture

These serious injuries are the least common simple pattern. Figure 4.20 shows the fracture pattern and mechanism of injury. Judet and Judet[7]

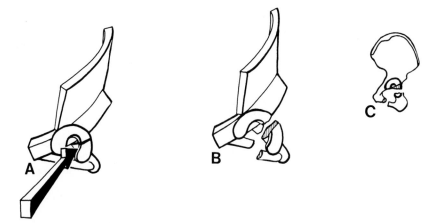

Figure 4.20.   Posterior column fracture. Posteroinferiorly directed force vector (*A*) fractures posterior column and inferior pubic ramus (*B* and *C*).

believe that these commonly result from a posteriorly directed force vector such as would occur from a blow to the knee with the hip flexed 95–100° and abducted 10–15°. The force vector is directed into the posterior column. Because of the massive size of the posterior column, a fracture through this region indicates a high energy load.

The fracture line runs through a segment of bone with a low section modulus, beginning close to the sciatic notch, extending downward and forward, and entering the acetabular notch. Thereafter it passes inferiorly through the obturator foramen and inferior pubic ramus.

Pelvic and acetabular fracture patterns have been classified according to the structural properties of the pelvis and how these relate to the various force vectors producing pelvic ring and acetabular disruption. This discussion has used the classifications of Pennal and Judet because they have achieved general acceptance and illustrate several important biomechanical principles. Unfortunately, as with most of our knowledge concerning pelvic biomechanics, these classifications are based mainly on clinical observation and await vigorous experimental verification. They are important for the surgeon because they allow him to analyze the radiological fracture patterns in a systematic manner, ascertain the nature of the forces involved, anticipate associated injuries, and plan a rational treatment protocol.

The simple biomechanical model of the pelvic, described here, combines the mechanical attributes of the ring, the column, and the triangle. This model does much to illustrate the biomechanics of the basic pelvic and acetabular fracture patterns.

This chapter draws attention to other engineering concepts such as viscoelasticity, stress concentration, section modulus, structural stability, and the parabolic stress distribution of forces across the hip joint.

References

1. BRAUS H: *Anatomie des Menschen*, vol. 1. Springer, Berlin, 1929.
2. CARRUTHERS FW, LOGUE RM: Treatment of fractures of the pelvis and their complications. *Am Acad Orthop Surg Inst Course Lect* 10:50–56, 1953.
3. DOMMISSE GF: Diametric fractures of the pelvis. *J Bone Joint Surg[Br]* 42B:432–443, 1960.
4. EVANS FG: *Stress and Strain in Bones. Their Relationship to Fractures and Osteogenesis.* Charles C Thomas, Springfield, Ill, 1957.
5. GERTZBEIN S, CHENOWETH DR: Occult fractures of the pelvis. *Clin Orthop* 128: 202–207, 1977.
6. HOWELL JB: Fractures of the pelvis. *Miss Doctor* 21:273, 1944.
7. JUDET R, JUDET J: Fractures of the acetabulum: classification and surgical approaches to open reduction. *J Bone Joint Surg* 46A:1615–1646, 1964.
8. KNIGHT RA, SMITH H: Central fractures of the acetabulum. *J Bone Joint Surg* 40A: 1–16, 1958.
9. LEIMBACKER ES: Injuries of the pelvis. *J Bone Joint Surg* 25:828–833, 1943.
10. McLAUGHLIN HL: *Trauma* pp. 477–494. WB Saunders, Philadelphia, 1959.
11. PAUWELS F: Die Bedeutung der Bauprinzipien des Stütz—und Bewegungsapparatus für die Beanspruchung der Röhrenknocken. Beitrag zur funktionellen Anatomie und Kausalen Morphologie der Stützapparatus. *Ztschr Anat Entwickle* 114:129–166, 1948.
12. PENNAL GF, SUTHERLAND G: Fractures of the Pelvis, 1961. (Motion picture available through the American Academy of Orthopedic Surgeons Film Library.)
13. PICK MP: A classification of fractures of the pelvis. *Proc R Soc Med* 48:96–98, 1955.
14. ROWE CR, LOWELL JD: Prognosis of fractures of the acetabulum. *J Bone Joint Surg* 43A:30–59, 1961.
15. SLATIS P, HUTTINEN VM: Double vertical fractures of the pelvis. *Acta Surg Scand* 138:799, 1972.
16. STEWARD MJ, MILFORD LW: Fracture dislocations of the hip. *J Bone Joint Surg* 36A:315–342, 1954.
17. SULLIVAN CR: Fractures of the pelvis. *Am Acad Orthop Surg Inst Course Lect* 18: 92–101, 1961.
18. WALLER Å: Dorsal acetabular fractures of the hip. *Acta Chir Scand* Suppl 205, 1955.

Questions—Chapter 4

1. Major pelvic ring disruption is most commonly associated with the following load configuration:
   a. tension
   b. bending
   c. compression
   d. torsion

2. Internal oblique views of the acetabulum (Judet) best delineate the following:
   a. anterior column and anterior lip of acetabulum
   b. anterior column and posterior lip of acetabulum
   c. posterior column and anterior lip of acetabulum
   d. posterior column and posterior lip of acetabulum
   e. all areas, equally

3. Which views give the most information about the displacement of pelvic ring fractures:
   a. AP and lateral view of pelvis
   b. three-quarter oblique views (Judet)
   c. inlet and tangential views of pelvis (Pennal).
   d. obstetrical inlet and outlet views
   e. any two views, provided they are taken at 45° angles from each other

4. In the erect posture the femoral-sacral arch is predominantly subjected to what load pattern:
   a. tension
   b. compression
   c. bending
   d. torsion

5. Which ligament is most important in providing pelvic ring stability:
   a. anterior sacroiliac ligament
   b. posterior sacroiliac ligament
   c. sacrospinous ligament
   d. sacrotuberous ligament
   e. inferior pubic ligament

6. What is the strongest portion of the pubic ligament complex:
   a. superior pubic ligament

    b. inferior pubic ligament
    c. anterior pubic ligament
    d. all portions share load equally

7. Mechanically the effect of having the stoutest ligaments about the periphery of the pelvic ring is to:
    a. increase stability
    b. decrease stability
    c. have no effect on stability

8. Which views give the most information in assessing acetabular fractures:
    a. AP and lateral views of pelvis
    b. three-quarter oblique views (Judet)
    c. inlet and tangential views of pelvis (Pennal)
    d. obstetrical inlet and outlet views
    e. any two views, provided they are taken at 45° angles from each other

9. In the standing position, which portion of the acetabulum is subjected to the greatest compression loads:
    a. anterior portion
    b. posterior portion
    c. dome portion
    d. central portion

10. External oblique views of the acetabulum best delineate the:
    a. anterior column and anterior lip of the acetabulum
    b. anterior column and posterior lip of the acetabulum
    c. posterior column and anterior lip of the acetabulum
    d. posterior column and posterior lip of the acetabulum

11. Which pelvic fracture pattern is most commonly associated with a bladder puncture:
    a. antroposterior compression
    b. ipsilateral compression
    c. contralateral compression
    d. ventrical shear

12. Which pelvic fracture pattern is the least stable:
    a. antroposterior compression
    b. ipsilateral compression
    c. contralateral compression
    d. vertical shear

13. The characteristics of a *vector* are:
    a. they involve high energy forces
    b. the forces must be of long duration
    c. it has a direction, magnitude and point of application
    d. none of the above

14. Mechanically, the effect of the acetabular notch is to:
    a. increase the strength of the acetabulum
    b. have no effect on the strength of the acetabulum
    c. weaken the area of the dome
    d. weaken the anterior and posterior margins of the acetabulum

15. According to Judet and Judet,[7] the forces across the hip joint:
    a. are evenly distributed over the articular surface
    b. are greater anteriorly than posteriorly
    c. are greatest at the dome
    d. follow a parabolic distribution

16. The fracture pattern expected to result from a blow to the anterior aspect of the iliac crest (directed posteriorly) would be
    a. bilateral pubic rami fractures (straddle fracture)
    b. hinge or open book fracture
    c. ipsilateral compression fracture
    d. contralateral compression fracture

17. The fracture pattern commonly associated with a pure lateral compression blow to the pelvis is:
    a. bilateral pubic rami fractures (straddle fracture)
    b. hinge or open book fracture
    c. ipsilateral compression fracture
    d. vertical shear fracture

18. With the hip flexed to 90° which position requires the greatest force to produce a fracture dislocation
    a. hip adducted 25°
    b. hip in neutral position
    c. hip adducted 15°
    d. hip adduction has no effect on the force required to produce a fracture

19. The Hinge or open book fracture pattern is most com-

monly associated with the disruption of the following ligament complex:

a. posterior sacroiliac ligament
b. anterior sacroiliac ligament
c. sacrotuberous ligament
d. sacrospino ligament

20. The load vector across the hip joint always passes through the:

a. greater trochanter
b. dome of the acetabulum
c. knee
d. center of the femoral head

Answers—Chapter 4: 1) c (see ''Type of Load''; Sullivan[17]); 2) b (Fig. 4.6); 3) c (Fig. 4.1); 4) b (Dommisse[5]); 5) b (see ''Ligamentous Supports''); 6) c (Dommisse[5]); 7) a (''Ligamentous-Supports''); 8) b (Fig. 4.6); 9) c (see ''Acetabulum''; Braus[2]; Pauwels[11]; Rowe and Lowell[14]); 10) c (Fig. 4.6); 11) b (Fig. 4.14); 12) d (see ''Vertical Shear''; Pennal and Sutherland[12]); 13) b (see ''Structural Properties''); 14) b (see ''Type of Load''); 15) d (Fig. 4.8); 16) b (Fig. 4.11); 17) c (Fig. 4.13); 18) a (Fig. 4.10); 19) b (see ''Pelvic Fractures''; 20) d (Fig. 4.9).

CHAPTER 5

Biomechanics of Spinal Injury

Dennis C. Evans

The prime objectives in the management of spinal cord injury are to prevent damage to nervous elements beyond that inflicted at the time of initial injury, preserve the remaining function, protect the injured tissues, and provide optimum conditions for recovery. In order to achieve these aims, it is essential to have an understanding of spinal biomechanics and to know how to apply them to the mechanism of the injury and the pathology of the lesions involving bone, soft tissue, and nervous tissue. In most instances, the mechanism of injury can be deduced by correlating clinical and radiological data with a knowledge of spinal lesions produced experimentally.

The effect of force applied to the spine depends upon certain inherent anatomical characteristics which enable it to withstand stress or which render it more vulnerable. These characteristics determine the degree of protection which is afforded to nerve tissue.

The bony spine has two important mechanical functions. It serves as a highly mobile central axis for the body and it protects the contents of the spinal canal. In the performance of these functions a delicate balance is maintained between stability and movement. To understand the biomechanics of spinal injury, the physician must think in terms of the forces producing the deformation (i.e., loads) and the structures resisting deformation (i.e., bony and soft tissue support). Stability depends upon the balance between applied load and the spinal bone and soft tissue support. Five factors determine the manner in which an injury will occur (see Ch. 1, "Long Bone Fracture Patterns"). Two of these factors arise from the physical properties of the object being injured and three from the characteristics of the applied load.

Object
   1. Material properties
   2. Structural properties
Load
   1. Type of load

2. Load rate
3. Magnitude of load

For the spine the *material properties* are primarily those of cancellous bone, ligaments, nuclear, and annular material; these are the basic building blocks of the spine. The *structural properties* dictate how size, shape, and location of the vertebrae, facets, ligaments, spinous, and transverse processes affect stability. The orthopedic literature contains extensive studies of these properties.

The loads to which an object can be subjected are combinations of tension, compression, bending, torsion, and shear. In clinical assessment, the loads are considered in terms of the movement they produce.

Movement	Load
Flexion	Bending
Extension	Bending
Lateral bending	Bending
Compression	Axial loading
Rotation	Torsion
Distraction	Tension
Translation	Shear

Thus, instead of talking about the stability of the spine to bending loads, we refer to *resistance* to flexion, extension, or lateral bending loads. This distinction is useful because we know that the spine has markedly different mechanical properties depending on the direction of bending (e.g., flexion *versus* lateral bending).

The *load rate* refers to how rapidly a load is applied to the spine. The spine (and most biological material) behaves quite differently when subjected to rapidly applied loads than when it is slowly deformed. As described in Chapter 1, any material that has this characteristic is called *viscoelastic*. Ligaments and the dynamic muscular support of the spine exhibit considerable viscoelastic behavior.

The *magnitude of load* refers to the quantity of force delivered. This energy is dissipated throughout the bony skeleton or through the soft tissue structures. If the magnitude exceeds the local breaking strength, the bone will fracture; if it exceeds the tensile strength of the ligament, it will rupture. Hence, the surgeon must always consider the magnitude of load in assessing the patient with a suspected spine injury. The sections to follow will describe how the interaction between the structural characteristics of the spine and the type of load to which it is subjected produces characteristic fracture patterns. The first section will discuss the anatomy of the spinal column and the biomechanics of a *single spinal segment* (spinal unit or motion segment). The next section will describe the mechanical characteristics of the various regions of the spine and how they relate to spinal injury. The final section will discuss the biomechanics of some common spinal injuries—whiplash and the seat belt injury and the biomechanics of stabilization following injury.

BIOMECHANICS AND ANATOMY OF SPINAL UNIT

The vertebral column is a multilinked system.[7] The individual links of the system, the 24 presacral vertebrae separated by 23 intervertebral discs, articulate with one another and are held together by a complicated arrangement of ligaments and muscles. On a lateral view the vertebral column is an S-shaped curve which is convex forward in the cervical and lumbar regions and convex posteriorly in the thoracic and sacral regions. In the erect posture the line of gravity intersects the presacral curves at the level of the 1st cervical, 7th cervical, 10th thoracic, and 2nd sarcal vertebrae. The body weight is more or less evenly distributed in front of and behind the gravity line. As a linked mechanical system, the great flexibility of the spinal column enables it to produce and accumulate moments of force, in addition to concentrating and transmitting forces it receives from other parts of the body.

The vertebral column can be considered as two subsystems: the vertebral bodies and intervertebral discs, which are the primary compression-resisting parts of the column; and the neural arches and associated ligaments, which are the tension-resisting parts.

The effect of forces acting on the spine can be clarified by analyzing the reaction of a complete spinal unit or motion segment to these forces.[33, 46] The anatomical characteristics of the unit are the major factors in determining resulting fracture patterns.

The spinal unit consists of two vertebrae joined by an intervertebral disc reinforced by the strong anterior longitudinal ligament[24] in front and by the posterior longitudinal ligament behind (compression resisting), and two posterior articulations with supporting capsule and interspinous ligaments (tension-resisting)[17] (Fig. 5.1). Direction of movement of the spine is determined mainly by the shape and position of the articulating processes of the diarthrodial joints (facet joints). Their orientation determines their mechanical importance.[45]

In the cervical spine the facets angle 45° to the frontal plane, the superior facets face upwards and backwards (Fig. 5.2A). This orientation permits marked mobility but renders this region vulnerable to injury.[13, 15]

In the thoracic spine the articular surface is nearly vertical. The superior facets face backwards and slightly laterally (Fig. 5.2B). The limited mobility afforded by the rib cage and short, strong interlaminar and interspinous ligaments adds to the stability of this region.

In the lumbar spine the articular facets are vertical and curve trans-

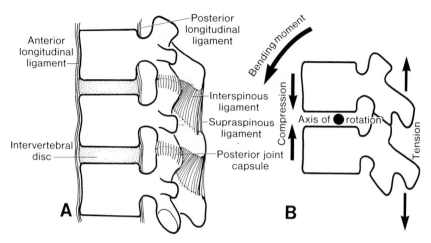

Figure 5.1. *A*, intervertebral ligaments. *B*, "spinal unit" or "motion segment."

versely, the superior facets look medially and backwards (Fig. 5.2*C*). The size and position of these facets contributes to local stability.

The ligamentum flavum has a high content of elastic fibers. In normal subjects it prestresses the intervertebral disc by a force ranging from 1500 g in the young to 400 g in the aged. Situated at a distance from the motion center of the disc, the interlaminar ligament is able to create an intradiscal pressure of about 0.70 kg/cm^2 in the upright position, at least in younger individuals.[25]

The interlaminar ligament appears to be a highly specialized tissue which protects nerve roots and also prestresses the disc, providing some intrinsic stability to the spine.

The following forces act on the spinal unit (Fig. 5.3): compression, bending (flexion and extension), torsion (rotation), tension (distraction), and shear (translation).

Compression (Axial Loading)

In the normal spine, as axial loading increases, the vertebral end plate bulges and squeezes blood out of the cancellous bone[33] (Fig. 5.4). The normal nucleus pulposus, however, is incompressible and maintains its shape. At loads greater than 500 lb,[30, 31] the end plate cracks and nuclear material is displaced into the vertebral body;[34] the result is disintegration of the disc. The normal elastic disc is stronger than bone and can withstand forces greater than the breaking point of the end plate.[41] There is no annular bulging until the disc loses its turgor, the end plate fractures, and the disc disintegrates. If the nucleus is no longer fluid and asymmetrical compression is applied, a different fracture pattern is produced

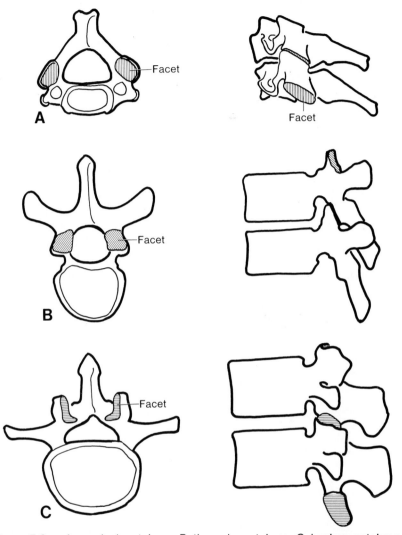

Figure 5.2.   *A*, cervical vertebrae. *B*, thoracic vertebrae. *C*, lumbar vertebrae.

(marginal plateau fracture or general collapse of the vertebrae). The nucleus retains its shape and turgor while it is normally hydrated but collapses and loses its normal mechanical properties if it becomes dehydrated (e.g., high incidence of compression fracture in the elderly).

Flexion (Bending)

Flexion or forward bending in the saggital plane increases loading (compression) of the vertebral body, and there is a concomitant increase

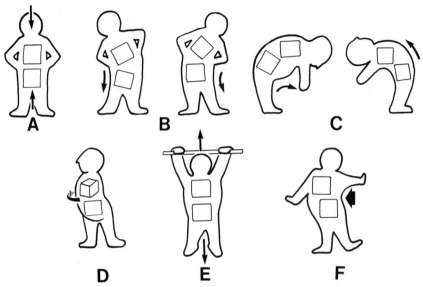

Figure 5.3. Forces acting on spinal unit. *A*, axial loading. *B* and *C*, bending. *D*, torsion. *E*, tension. *F*, shear.

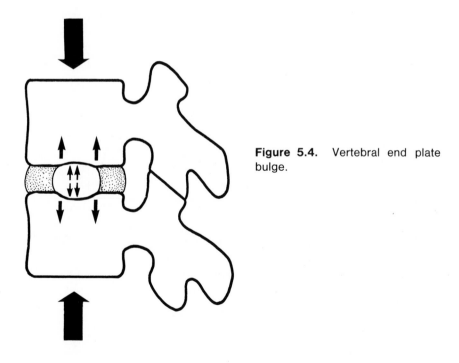

Figure 5.4. Vertebral end plate bulge.

in tension of the posterior ligament complex, particularly the longer interspinous ligament. Pressure at the fulcrum (anterior part of vertebral body) is three to four times greater than tension on the posterior ligament where the breaking point is about 400 lb,[3] a figure which exceeds the breaking point of the end plate. Thus, the vertebral body is crushed before the posterior ligament ruptures. Clinically, such an injury produces a variable degree of wedge compression in which the posterior interspinous ligaments remain intact (Fig. 5.5).

Extension (Bending)

Extension or backward bending compresses the posterior elements and increases tension anteriorly; however, crush fracture of the neural arch occurs first and there is little or no effective tension at the anterior longitudinal ligament (Fig. 5.6). There is no detectable alteration in the shape of the nucleus pulposus and no significant posterior bulge on extension. After denucleation, however, there is excessive mobility and annular bulge posteriorly.[33]

Rotation (Torsion)

The intervertebral disc, joint, and ligaments are resistant to compression, distraction, and bending but are vulnerable to rotation. Rotation

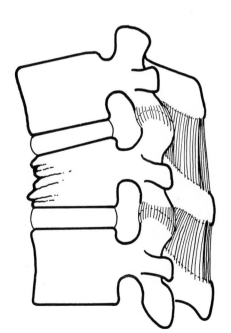

Figure 5.5. Wedge compression fracture with intact posterior ligament complex.

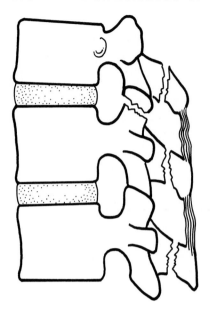

Figure 5.6. Posterior arch fracture following extension.

produces disruption of the ligaments and subsequent dislocation. If the spine is held in flexion and a rotational force applied, the posterior ligament, joint capsules, and posterior longitudinal ligament tear in that order and permit dislocation. There may be an associated fracture of the vertebral body, depending upon the amount of associated compression force (Fig. 5.7). Similarly, the anterior longitudinal ligament will rupture first if rotation is applied when the spine is in extension.[33]

When the nucleus pulposus has lost its turgor, these effects produce intervertebral displacement and subluxation more easily. The articular process may fracture, depending on the degree of associated flexion at the time of rotation. The clinical lesion is either a dislocation or fracture dislocation and both are unstable because of the ligament disruption.

Of all the loading mechanisms to which it is subjected, the spine is least able to resist rotation, particularly in the cervical and thoracolumbar regions.

Distraction (Tension)

As an isolated or dominant force, distraction or tension is uncommon, but it does occur in patients wearing a lap seat belt at the time of injury. On sudden deceleration the body is flexed over the restraining lap belt. The point of contact between the belt and the abdominal wall becomes the axis around which flexion occurs (Fig. 5.8). All portions of the spinal column are posterior to the flexion axis; therefore, the entire vertebral

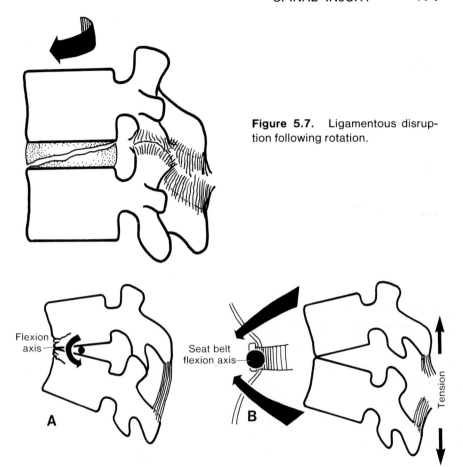

Figure 5.7.   Ligamentous disruption following rotation.

Figure 5.8.   *A*, flexion axis of spinal unit. *B*, forward movement of flexion axis to point of contact of seat belt against abdominal wall, resulting in tension stress or distraction to the spine posterior to the axis.

body and the neural arches are exposed to tensile stress. Disruption due to distraction may occur through soft tissue, bone or a combination.[39]

Distraction (tension) is more common in a region of the spinal unit opposite to an area under compression. As previously described, in hyperflexion the vertebral body is under compression while the interspinous ligament complex is under tension.

Translation (Shear)

Translation can occur in combination with other loading mechanisms and may be a major component in fracture dislocation of the thoracolumbar spine. The injury is usually associated with a high incidence of neurological deficit.

Except in the experimental situation, force applied to the spine seldom acts in a single plane; it is usually a composite of forces in which one or other is dominant.

The following force patterns can produce spinal injury: compression, flexion rotation, extension rotation, and distraction.

The effect of these forces in the different segments of the spinal column varies considerably because of anatomical differences in the particular region. The next section will examine the effects of these forces and the lesions they produce in the various regions.

CERVICAL SPINE

The cervical spine has a high degree of mobility and consequently a high susceptibility to injury. The total range of motion in cervical flexion and extension is 127°, lateral bending 73°, and rotation 142°.[8]

The axis of motion, or the "line of zero velocity," passes along the posterior margins of the vertebral bodies. Table 5.1 and Figure 5.9 show the average range of flexion and extension at each vertebral level. There is greater movement during extension than during flexion at only two levels, C6-7 and C7-T1. At C5-6 the average range of flexion is 15° and extension, 3°. The limited extension at this point may account for the vulnerability of this region to extension flexion and extension injury.[1]

Similarly limited flexion at the C6-7 and C7-T1 renders the cervical spine vulnerable at these levels in flexion injuries.

Table 5.1 Flexion and Extension at Each Vertebral Level

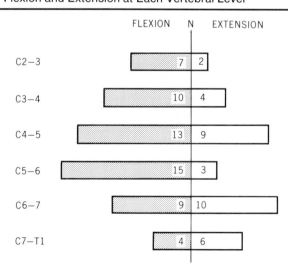

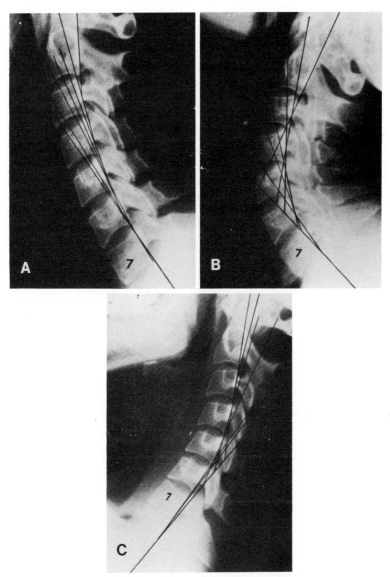

Figure 5.9.   Lateral roentgenograms of the cervical spine in neutral (*A*), extension (*B*), flexion (*C*). The inked lines indicate the angulation of each cervical vertebra in relation to the first thoracic vertebra.

ATLANTOAXIAL REGION

The atlantoaxial region has a specific pattern of injury by virtue of its unique anatomical features.

Compression

Compression of this region results from a direct force on the top of the head. The force is transmitted through the condyles of the occiput and the lateral masses of the atlas, which are forced apart (Fig. 5.10*A*). Fracture occurs at the weak points of the ring anteriorly and posteriorly[42] (Fig. 5.10*B*). There is widening of the interval between the lateral masses.[19] Both lateral masses come to overhang the lateral edge of the facets of the axis (Fig. 5.11). This injury, the Jefferson fracture, must be distinguished from ligamentous laxity, which produces overlap to the side of the lateral flexion, either left or right (Fig. 5.12). If the transverse ligament remains intact, there is no forward shift of the arch (Fig. 5.13) and, as a consequence, the cord is less vulnerable.

Flexion Rotation

Flexion rotation occurs when rotation is applied to the neck in a flexed

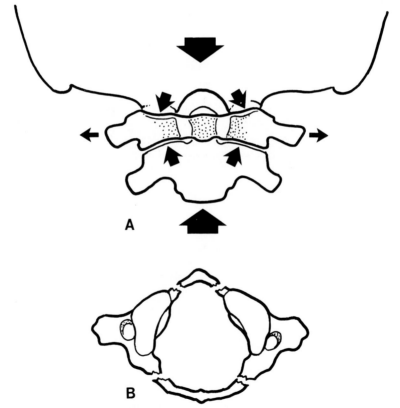

Figure 5.10.   *A*, compression force to atlas vertebrae. *B*, fracture of the C1 ring at the weak points anteriorly and posteriorly (Jefferson fracture).

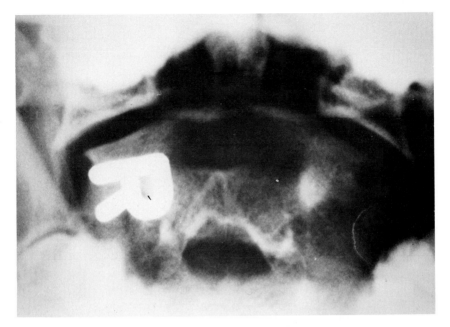

Figure 5.11. Roentgenogram of Jefferson fracture.

position. As shown experimentally, rotation disrupts the supporting ligaments and permits a forward shift on flexion. The resulting lesion is either subluxation with a rupture of the transverse ligament or a fracture of the odontoid.

Subluxation (Rupture of Transverse Ligament)

In flexion rotation, the transverse ligament which embraces the odontoid is torn and the atlas shifts forward, creating a gap between the arch of the atlas and the odontoid (Fig. 5.14A). Rupture of this ligament renders the cord vulnerable to compression by the odontoid (Fig. 5.14B).

Fielding et al.[9] have shown experimentally that the force required to rupture the transverse ligament is a mean of 111 Kilopond (kilogram force, kgf) under rapid loading and a mean of 72 kgf under slow loading, with a mean of 84 kgf for the combined group. After failure of the transverse ligament, the force necessary to produce further anterior shift, up to the end point of 12 mm, ranged from 20 to 120 kgf (mean 72). The alar ligament stretched but did not break during the 12 mm displacement.

Radiologically, a gap of 3 mm between the odontoid and the arch is within normal limits. In children this gap may be as wide as 4 mm. In the adult, if the displacement is 3 to 5 mm, one may conclude that the transverse ligament has ruptured, and if the displacement exceeds 5 mm,

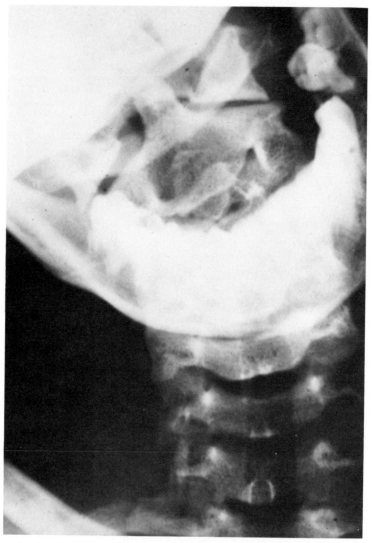

Figure 5.12. Roentgenogram showing lateral mass overhang due to capsular laxity.

the transverse ligament has ruptured and the accessory ligaments are stretched or deficient.[10]

To demonstrate the gap radiologically, it may be necessary to take lateral projections with the head and neck in flexion and extension (Fig. 5.15). The space available for the cord is the narrowest distance between the posterior edge of the vertebral body and the anterior edge of the

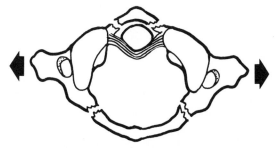

Figure 5.13.   Jefferson fracture with intact transverse ligament.

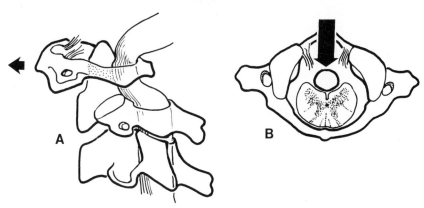

Figure 5.14.   *A*, forward displacement of C1 on C2 due to ligamentous disruption (transverse ligament). *B*, transverse ligament rupture showing cord vulnerability.

posterior vertebral arch. This space should be greater than 14 mm from C1 to C7. The width of the odontoid is approximately equal to the space occupied by the cord at the C1 level and is therefore a guide to the space available for the cord.[10]

If the space available for the cord is less than the width of the odontoid, the safety of the cord may be compromised.

Fracture of Odontoid

The ligament may remain intact but the base of the odontoid may fracture (Fig. 5.16*A*). The transverse ligament embracing the odontoid remains intact; consequently, the odontoid moves forward and backward on flexion and extension. In this circumstance the cord is protected from the odontoid and is less vulnerable than in subluxation, where the ligament is ruptured.

Radiologically, the lesion can be demonstrated on the anteroposterior "open mouth" and lateral projections (Fig. 5.16*B*, *C*). However, it may

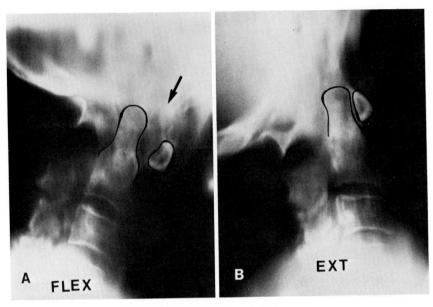

Figure 5.15.   Roentgenograms showing (*A*) relationship of the odontoid to the anterior arch of the atlas (normal position), and (*B*) gap between the odontoid and the anterior arch of the atlas (transverse ligament rupture).

be necessary to perform tomograms to show the lesion, which may be obscured, particularly on the lateral projection (Fig. 5.16*B–D*).

Fracture Dislocation C2–3

The posterior ligament complex is disrupted and allows C2 to shift forward on C3. There may be associated fracture of body and facets of C3.

Extension Rotation

The unsupported head perches on the mobile cervical spine is subject to sudden deflection as in acceleration-deceleration situations or in falls when the chin, forehead, or vertex strikes on obstacle. Extension is the dominant force but to it may be added elements of compression, distraction, and rotation. Owing to the limitation of extension imposed by the bony elements posteriorly, the fractures which result may involve:

1. The arch of C1 or C2 (Figs. 5.17 and 5.18).
2. Pedicles of C2 (Fig. 5.19).
3. Traumatic spondylolisthesis of the axis (Fig. 5.20). Garber[12, 14] used this term to denote a fracture of the pedicles of C2 with displacement of the body of the axis. The dens remains intact. The axis breaks symmet-

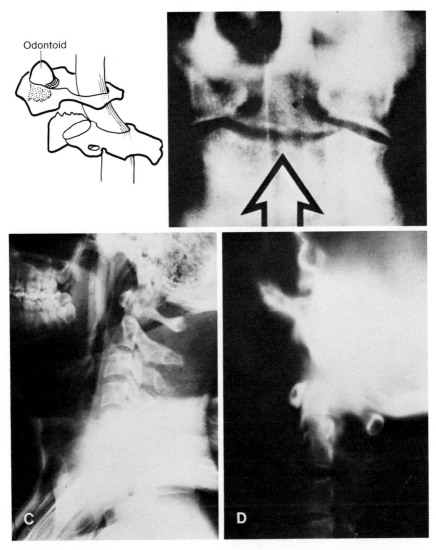

Figure 5.16. *A*, forward shift of C1 on C2 due to fracture of the odontoid. Roentgenograms of (*B*) odontoid fracture (open-mouth view) and (*C*) lateral view of odontoid fracture. (*D*) tomogram showing fracture of the odontoid.

rically across the pedicles or lateral masses, and the fracture may extend across the posterior part of the body. The presence of the foramina transversaria make the weakest part of the bony ring of the axis (Fig. 5.21). This region is the point of greatest leverage between the extended "cervico-cranium"—skull, atlas, dens and body of the axis—and the

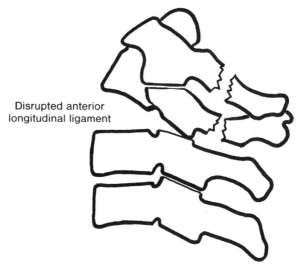

Disrupted anterior
longitudinal ligament

Figure 5.17. Extension fracture dislocation of C1 and C2.

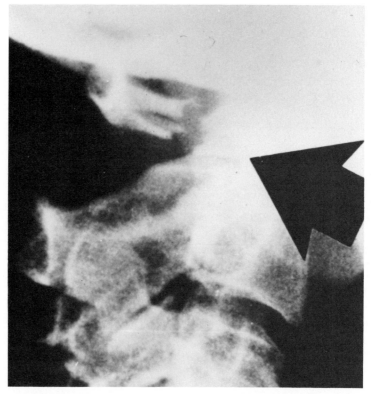

Figure 5.18. Roentgenogram of fracture of arch of atlas.

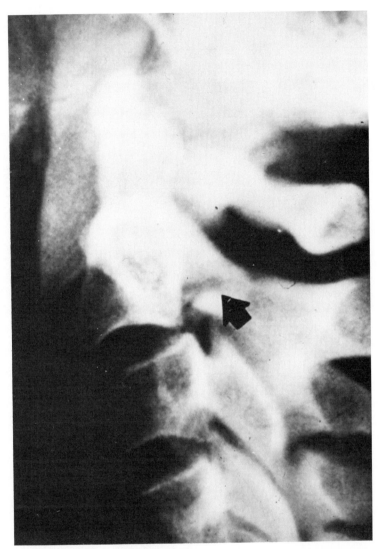

Figure 5.19. Roentgenogram of fracture of pedical of C2.

relatively fixed lower cervical spine; the neural arch of the axis is anchored to the latter by the inferior facets, spinous processes, and strong nuchal muscles[2, 50] (Fig. 5.22). The weight of the head falls forward and produces a shift of the axis, but its movement is limited by the intact posterior interspinous ligaments. This clinical picture erroneously suggests a flexion injury when the true mechanism of injury is *extension with compression* (axial loading). This lesion must be distinguished from a lesion which has a similar appearance but is produced by the different mechanism, exten-

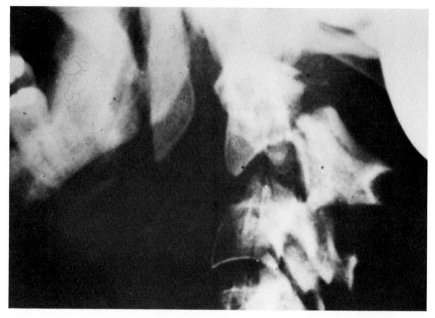

Figure 5.20. Roentgenogram of extension—traumatic spondylolisthesis of the axis.

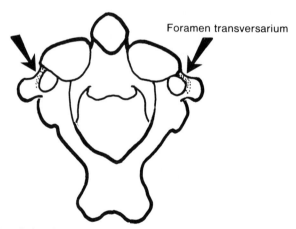

Foramen transversarium

Figure 5.21. Axis showing foramen transversarium. (The pedicles are the thinnest part of the bony ring which is weakened by the foramen transversarium.)

sion, and distraction. The term "hangman's fracture" has been applied to both lesions but should be reserved for the extension-distraction lesion.

Extension and compression (Fig. 5.23) are produced by a fall in which the chin, forehead, or vertex strikes an obstacle or by head-on collisions

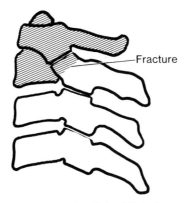

—Fracture

Figure 5.22. The region of stress (pedicle C2) between the extending cervi-cocranium (*hatched*) and the relatively fixed lower cervical region.

in which the head strikes the interior of a vehicle. Neurological injury is rare, possibly because the spinal canal is sufficiently wide at this level to accommodate some movement of the fragments which tend to separate and widen the canal. Associated midcervical injuries and fractures of the spinous processes, which are sometimes seen, suggest that there has been considerable compression.

Extension and Distraction (Fig. 5.24) of the upper cervical spine follows violent extension when the rapidly moving body is suddenly restrained under the chin or across the front of the neck. This combination of events occurs in judicial hanging with a submental knot and "long drop" and can occur following restraint by a loose diagonal seat belt in a head-on accident.[36, 51]

Distraction is a more violent injury than compression and thus there is a greater likelihood of neurological sequelae following direct injury to the cord.

Although reports of the lesion do not mention rotation as a component in this injury, this element is probably a factor in instances of anterior longitudinal ligament disruption, with the possible exception of that which occurs during hanging.

C3–C7 REGION

The same forces act in this region but the pattern of injury is different because of the anatomical features.

Compression

The cervical spine has a natural lordosis, but as the neck moves from the extended (lordotic) (Fig. 5.25C) to the flexed position (Fig. 5.25A), it reaches a point where the vertebrae are in vertical alignment (Fig. 5.25B).

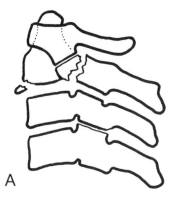

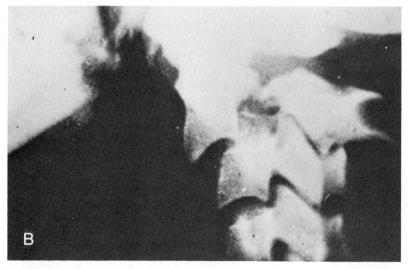

Figure 5.23. *A*, traumatic spondylolisthesis of axis (extension compression). *B*, roentgenogram of traumatic spondylolisthesis of axis.

In this position a compression force will produce a Burst fracture of the vertebral body, most commonly of C5 or C6. The force results in explosive disruption of the vertebrae; the posterior portion explodes into the canal but is restrained by the posterior longitudinal ligament, which may or may not be breached. Radiologically, there is no obvious abnormality on anteroposterior view. Lateral projection reveals that the vertebral body is comminuted and that the posterior inferior portion is protruding into the canal (Fig. 5.26). Considering the magnitude of the neurological injury in some cases, the overall radiological appearance is unimpressive. The maximum damage occurs at the time of injury. The dura remains intact anteriorly and posteriorly, but there may be extensive contusion and cord

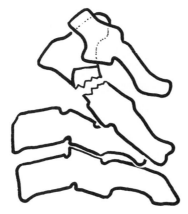

Figure 5.24. Hangman's fracture (extension distraction).

disruption in patients with a neurological deficit (Fig. 5.27). More commonly the neurological damage is extensive with quadriplegia, but in some cases it is minimal or nil.

This fracture may be associated with an anterior cord syndrome in which neurological deficit involves the anterior portion of the cord with sparing of the posterior columns. This lesion is considered to be stable as the posterior ligament complex remains intact. However, the comminuted vertebral body is subject to axial loading and further compression.

Flexion Rotation

This implies a force applied to the head, producing both flexion and rotation. Rotation disrupts the ligaments, i.e., interspinous, capsular, posterior longitudinal,[29] disc and anterior longitudinal ligament, in that order. The degree of disruption will vary according to the force. If the flexion component is great, the facets will disengage and permit dislocation with forward shift. When the flexion is of lesser degree, the facets will be incompletely disengaged and the facets will be fractured.

Subluxation

Subluxation occurs following flexion rotation that is insufficient to produce dislocation. Spontaneous reduction occurs when the neutral position is resumed. Routine radiographs may fail to show the lesion (Fig. 5.28A); however, flexion-extension views will show the inferior facet riding up on the superior facet of the vertebrae below, (Fig. 5.28B) following disruption of the interspinous ligament. If the disruption is marked, the tell-tale gap between the spinous processes will be evident on the antero-posterior (AP) view (Fig. 5.28C). This sign indicates an unstable segment and a potentially hazardous lesion. Subsequently, a force of lesser degree

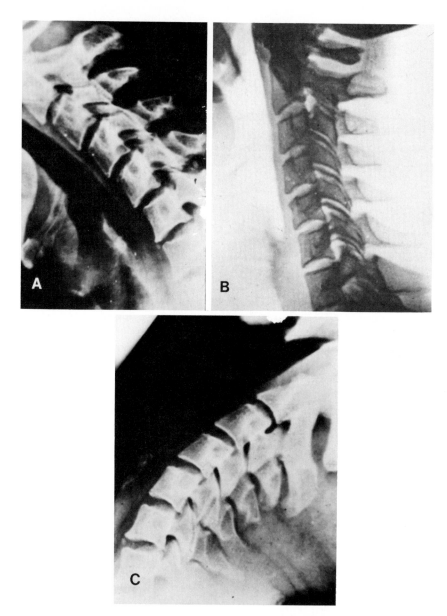

Figure 5.25.   Lateral roentgenogram of the cervical spine showing the position of the vertebrate in the extended (*C*) and flexed positions (*A*). *B*, compression force to the vertebrate in this position results in a burst fracture.

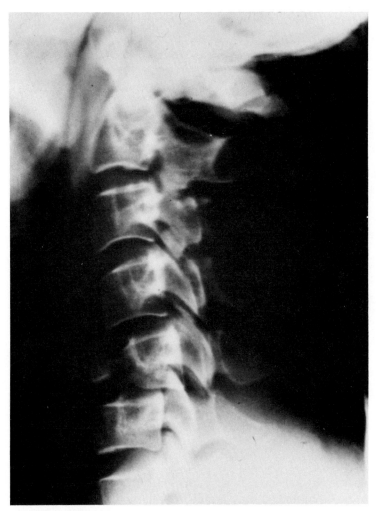

Figure 5.26.   Lateral roentgenogram showing burst fracture.

than that which produced the initial injury may disrupt the scar tissue
and complete the dislocation, with disastrous consequences.

If extension produces no spontaneous reduction, the patient may have
a "perched facet" (Fig. 5.29A). In the case illustrated here the inferior
facet of C5 is perched on the superior facet of C6. Exploration demonstrated a crack involving the tip of the superior facet of C6 which was not
evident radiologically. However, the gap between the C5 and C6 spinous
processes on the AP view indicated that the lesion was unstable (Fig.
5.29B).

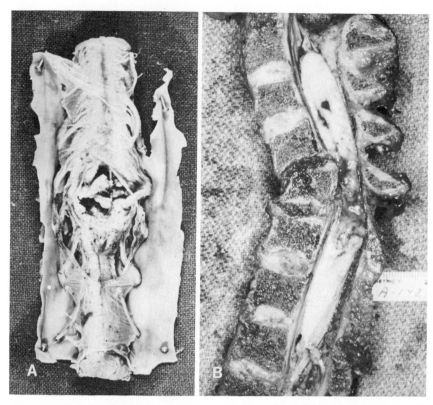

Figure 5.27.   *A*, specimen showing cord disruption from burst fracture. *B*, saggital section of cervical spine showing cord disruption from burst fracture.

Dislocation

When the flexion force is great enough to disengage the facets, the dislocation so produced may result in unilateral locked facet, bilateral locked facet, fracture dislocation, or wedge compression.

Unilateral Locked Facet. One facet disengages and displaces while the opposite side remains in position. Radiologically, on the AP projection the spinous processes above the dislocation are out of alignment with the spinous processes below the level of the lesion (Fig. 5.30*A*). The displacement is to the same side of the midline as the locked facet. On lateral projection the facets below the dislocation are superimposed and seen as one, whereas above the lesion the facets are offset and seen one in front of the other, giving a "bow-tie"[5] appearance (Fig. 5.30*B* and *C*). The displacement of the body is evident, but the shift is less than half the width of the vertebral body and will not increase with further movement.

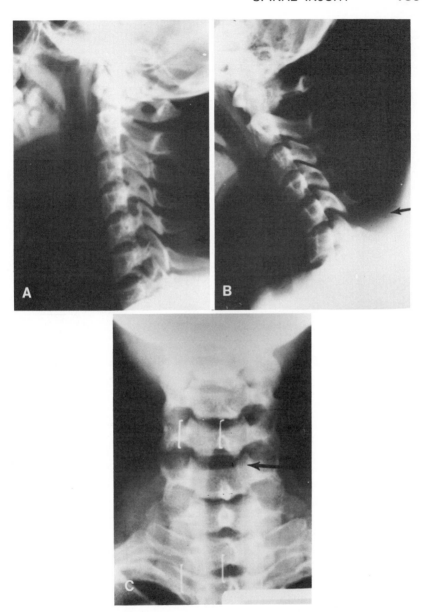

Figure 5.28.   Roentgenograms showing lateral views of subluxation at C5–6 (A) but not evident as the vertebra are in the reduced position, and subluxation at C5–6 (B)—wide gap posteriorly evident on flexion of the spine. C, AP view of gap at the C5–6 level due to posterior ligament disruption.

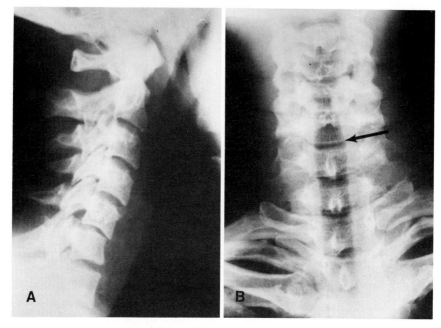

Figure 5.29. Roentgenograms showing lateral view of "perched facet" (A). Inferior facet of C5 perched on superior facet of C6 (due to a fracture at the tip of superior facet C6 but not evident radiologically). B, AP view of gap between spinous processes at C5–C6 due to ligamentous disruption and instability.

Bilateral Locked Facet. Both facets disengage and are seen as bilateral locked facets. On AP projection the spinous processes are in alignment above and below the level of the lesion. However, the gap between the spinous processes is always increased because of the ligamentous disruption (Fig. 5.31A). This change indicates instability of the spinal unit. The lesion is obvious on lateral projection because more than half the diameter of the body is displaced and this may increase in further flexion (Fig. 5.31B).

Fracture Dislocation. Fracture dislocation develops following flexion rotation, in which the dominant rotation force is associated with incomplete flexion. The facet is usually fractured and there is some degree of vertebral body compression. This lesion is grossly unstable but may readily reduce when the supine position is assumed. If this happens, the surgeon may not appreciate the unstable nature of the lesion. Lateral radiographs reveal a fracture dislocation with the fracture of the vertebral body (Fig. 5.32A). The AP view shows the telltale gap between the spinous processes at the level of dislocation (Fig. 5.32B).

It is imperative that all the vertebrae be seen in both views. Failure to

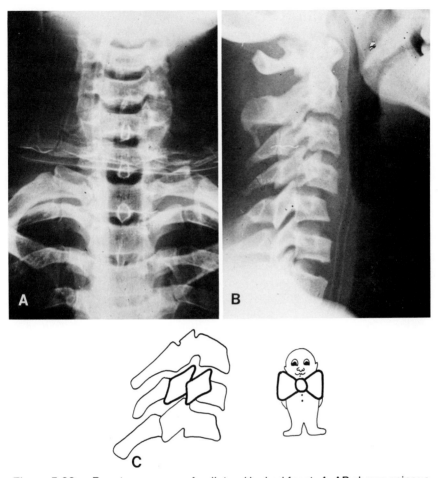

Figure 5.30.   Roentgenograms of unilateral locked facet. *A*, AP shows spinous processes offset to the left at C4 and proximally. The C5 spinous process and those distally are midline and in alignment. *B*, lateral view shows the facets at C4 and proximal are offset and exhibit a "bow tie" appearance. The facets below are in alignment and appear as one. The vertebral shift is less than 50% of the vertebral body. *C*, diagram of "bow tie" appearance of the offset facets.

demonstrate all the cervical vertebrae radiologically may result in a lesion of the lower level cervical region being missed (Fig. 5.33*A*). All the vertebrae can be exposed by pulling the arms distally at the sides or forwards as in the swimmer's position (Fig. 5.33*B*). The gap on the AP view should draw attention to a lesion which may remain undetected on the lateral view (Fig. 5.33*C*). However, if the spinous process is fractured and floating, the gap may not be evident. It may be necessary to make

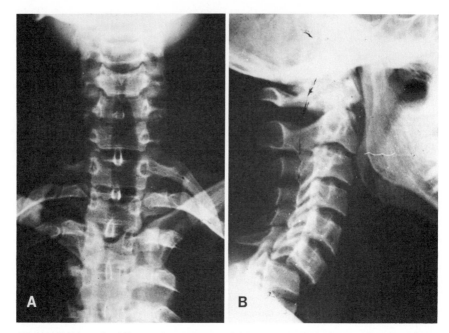

Figure 5.31. *A*, AP roentgenogram of bilateral locked facet. Gap between spinous processes at C6–C7. Processes are in alignment. *B*, lateral view of dislocation at C6–C7. Displacement more than 50% of vertebral body.

tomograms when the areas cannot be visualized and the surgeon suspects a fracture dislocation (Fig. 5.34).

Wedge Compression. When flexion is the dominant force and there is no significant rotation, the injury will produce a wedge compression fracture of the vertebral body. The posterior ligament complex remains intact. This injury is usually unassociated with a neurological deficit.

Extension Rotation

Fracture Dislocation

Extension rotation force produces a fracture dislocation. Careful examination will often reveal abrasions or lacerations on the patient's face or forehead, indicating the direction of force and suggesting the extension mechanism. The rotation element produces ligamentous disruption of the anterior longitudinal ligament first and, in order posteriorly, of the posterior longitudinal, capsular, and interspinous ligaments. Owing to the apposition of the bony elements, the spinous process fractures near its base, and the injury may involve fracture of the articular processes which, because of the compression, come to lie in a more horizontal plane.

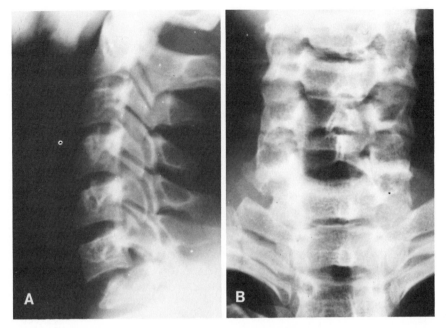

Figure 5.32.   Roentgenograms showing lateral view of fracture dislocation at C6–C7 (*A*), and AP view of fracture dislocation C6–C7 (*B*) with gap between spinous processes due to posterior disruption.

Concurrent disruption of the anterior longitudinal ligament produces a small avulsion fracture at the inferior margin of the vertebrae (Fig. 5.35). Although the spinous process is fractured, the interspinous ligament remains intact. In the upright or prone position the weight of the head carries the upper vertebrae forward but this movement is limited by the posterior ligaments (Fig. 5.36). A lateral radiograph may show a slight forward shift and may erroneously suggest a flexion-type injury. However, the presence of facial abrasions, the transverse position of the facets and spinous processes, and the avulsed fragment anteriorly should suggest the true nature of the lesion. The associated neurological lesion may be minimal or extensive.

Central Cord Syndrome[32, 37]

Occasionally a patient may present with an extensive neurological lesion but no evidence of an associated radiological bony injury. Such a lesion can be due to a central cervical cord injury. The syndrome is characterized by a disproportionately greater motor impairment of the upper than of the lower extremities and is combined with bladder dysfunction and varying degrees of sensory loss below the level of the lesion.

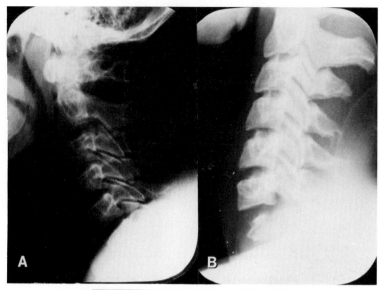

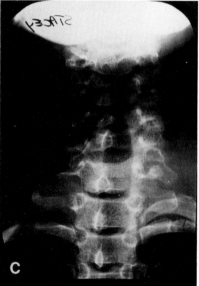

Figure 5.33. *A,* lateral roentgenogram; lower cervical vertebrae not visualized. *B,* fracture dislocation at C6–C7 revealed on visualization of the lower cervical vertebrae by pulling the arms distally or forwards. *C,* AP roentgenogram; gap between C6–C7 indicates unstable lesion present, and subsequently visualized on lateral view by exposing lower vertebrae (see Fig. 5.42*B*).

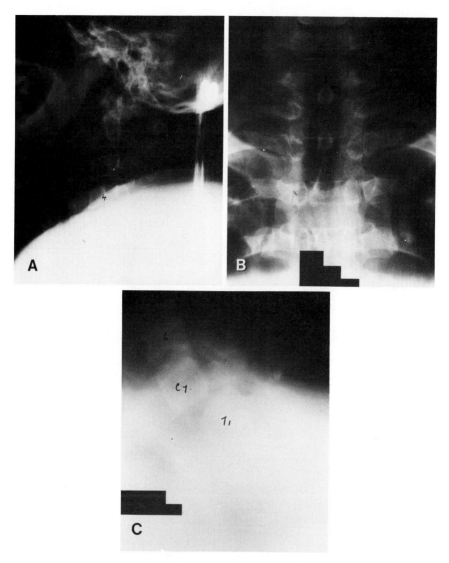

Figure 5.34.   *A*, lateral roentgenogram of cervical spine of 300-lb male with bull neck. A satisfactory lateral radiograph could not be obtained. *B*, AP view of lower cervical region appears normal. Fracture dislocation was present at C7–T1, but the gap was not evident as the spinous process was fractured and floating (revealed at operation). Lesion revealed by tomography. *C*, tomogram of C7–T1 showing dislocation.

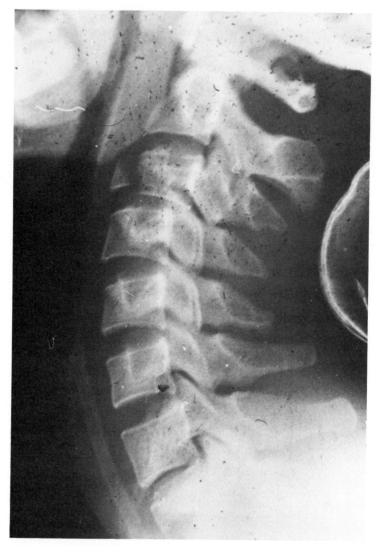

Figure 5.35.   Lateral roentgenogram showing extension fracture dislocation of C3 with an avulsion fragment of the anterior inferior portion of C3.

Abrasion of the forehead should suggest the mechanism of injury, namely extension, which is frequently associated. The lesion is more common in a cervical spine that exhibits posterior spur formation.

During extension, the ligamentum flavum bulges forward, further reducing the AP diameter of the canal and producing an AP compressive force. The net result is a central cord hemorrhage with an area of surrounding edema. It has been shown that the force acting in the central

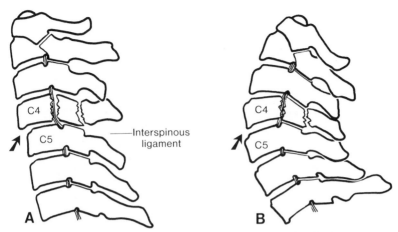

Figure 5.36. *A*, forward shift of C4, but flexion limited by the intact posterior ligaments. Forward shift erroneously suggests a flexion injury. *B*, vertebrate in the reduced position.

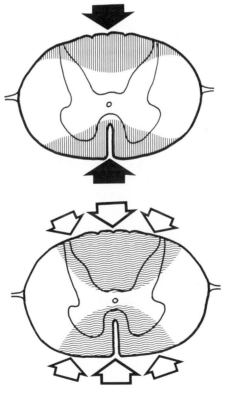

Figure 5.37. Anteroposterior compression forces on the cord.

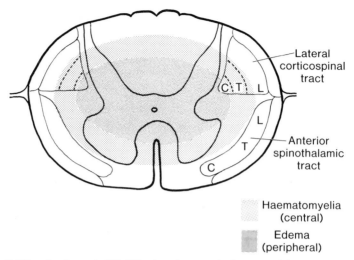

Figure 5.38.   Lesion at C5–C6 showing central area of hematomyelia and peripheral area of edema. *C*, cervical; *T*, thoracic; *L*, lumbar.

portion of the cord is five times greater than that acting in the lateral peripheral area (Fig. 5.37). Maximal damage is due to the central area of hemorrhage, the surrounding area of edema being capable of recovery (Fig. 5.38). The corticospinal tracts carrying motor impulses have an apex which points centrally; in these tracts the area supplying the hands and upper limbs is most central, followed by that supplying the trunk and lower limbs. The maximal damage occurs in the apical region and extends peripherally, depending on the degree of hematomyelia and edema. The spinothalamic tracts carrying pain and touch lie peripheral and may be spared or, because of the peripheral arrangement, may be impinged upon by edema or hematomyelia in an irregular manner, resulting in no sensory deficit or an irregular pattern. Recovery of function takes place in the reverse order; the most peripherally placed areas recover first, and the residual deficit, if any, is due to central damage.

Radiographic Pointers

The lesions produced by forces acting on the cervical spine can usually be demonstrated by standard radiographic projections, i.e., anteroposterior, lateral, oblique, and flexion extension stress views. However, it is also important to visualize all the vertebrae, to recognize soft tissue shadows (prevertebral hematoma) and to look for the interspinous gap which indicates instability.

An additional projection, "the pillar view,"[43] defines the area between the superior and inferior facets which may harbor a fracture and not be

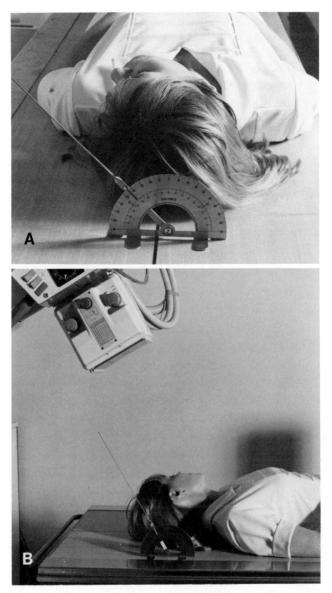

Figure 5.39. Radiographic technique to demonstrate pillar view. Head tilted 45° to the left to show the right pillar (*A*), while the tube is tilted 35° caudad (*B*).

revealed using standard projections. This technique positions the patient supine with his head turned 45° to the left to show the right pillar and, vice versa, to show the left while the tube is tilted 35° caudad (Fig. 5.39). Figure 5.40 shows a near normal lateral radiograph, whereas the pillar view shows a distinct area of increased density which is due to the 180° rotation of the bone mass bearing the superior and inferior facet.

Tomography may be required to demonstrate areas which cannot be visualized by these techniques. Figure 5.41 shows a fracture dislocation at the C7–T1 level in a 300-lb man with a short "bull" neck which could not be demonstrated using standard projections.

Cineradiography may help to demonstrate abnormal mobility and is especially useful in the atlantoaxial region.

THORACIC SPINE

The kyphotic thoracic spine supports the lordotic cervical spine and itself is supported by the lordotic lumbar spine. This region has several distinguishing features. The superior facets face posteriorly and slightly laterally, and the inferior facets are reciprocal. The size of the osseous segments increases caudally, and the segments have flat superior and inferior surfaces. The lamina tend to shingling, and the short thick ligamentum flavum limits rotation and bending. Finally, the thinner discs and short interspinous ligaments increase this limitation. The combination of the oblique orientation of the facets and the short intersegmental

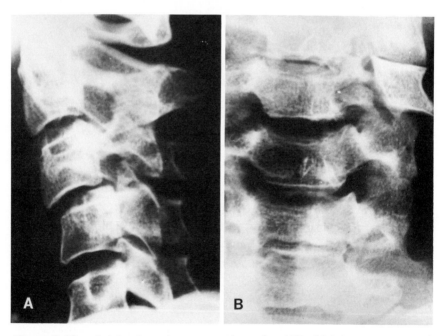

Figure 5.40. *A*, lateral roentgenogram shows facet tilt of C4, but true nature of lesion is not clear. *B*, pillar view clearly demonstrates facets rotated 180°. (Increased density indicates rotations.)

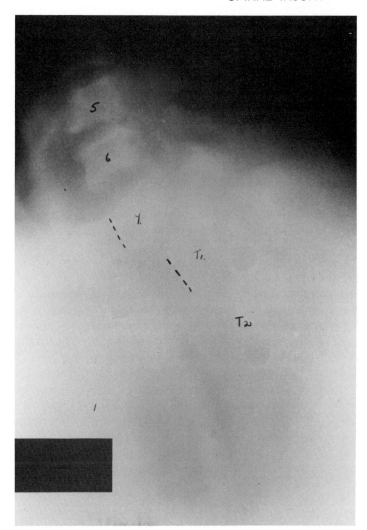

Figure 5.41.   Tomogram shows fracture dislocation at C7–T1 which could not be demonstrated by usual techniques.

ligaments produces a greater restriction of movement in the thoracic region than elsewhere.

An additional feature makes this region unique: the ribs function as stabilizing outriggers, restricting lateral flexion and extension. The parallel arrangement of the ribs, however, decreases this resistance to torsion. Rotation is free, and 70% of the thoracolumbar range occurs within the thoracic region. On the other hand, because they lie in the frontal plane, the articular facets allow relatively free motion around all three spatial axes. The upper and lower portions of the thoracic spine behave quite differently and have certain traits in common with the adjacent region. Between these two areas is a homogeneous section characterized by limited movement and therefore stability. The extrinsic stability is provided by the trunk and back musculature. The action of the thoracic and abdominal musculature increases the intracavitary pressure and permits the thoracic spine to withstand forces that otherwise might result in injury.[20, 23]

The *10th* to the *12th* thoracic vertebrae form a transition zone between two regions with high torsional stiffness (the 10th thoracic vertebrae and above articulate with the rib cage and the lumbar spine has inherently high torsional stiffness). The application of sudden torsional moments, as might develop within the spinal column during a fall, is likely to result in the intermediate zone absorbing a great deal of energy since rotation would be greatest at these levels. Clinically, the transitional region is a common site for spinal injury.[21]

Experimental removal of the posterior elements increases the amount of motion in flexion, extension, and axial rotation.[46] Clinically, this may occur in circumstances where the posterior elements lose support through injury, and this increases both the range of motion and the magnitude of load.

Motion is greater in the direction of loading than in the other directions except during axial compression, which produces nearly 50% more translation in the horizontal direction than in the axial direction.[27, 28]

Bending moment and axial compression forces produce compressive normal stresses which are additive at the anterior portion of the thoracic vertebrae. This is probably the most reasonable explanation of the high incidence of vertebral fracture in the thoracic region.[26]

Flexion

The thoracic spine is subject mainly to the force of flexion, flexion rotation, and, less commonly, lateral flexion. This section of the spine resists extension. The distance between the flexion axis and the tip of the spinous process is three to four times greater than the distance between the axis and the anterior margin of the vertebral body. Therefore, when exposed to flexion stress, the anterior portion of the vertebral body experiences a compression load that is three to four times greater than the tensile load falling upon the spinous process and supraspinous ligaments. Thus, hyperflexion produces a wedge-shaped fracture of the vertebral body but never produces posterior element avulsion or ligament rupture[35] (Fig. 5.42). Crushing of the anterior body allows energy dissipation and dampens weak loads, so that flexion alone cannot generate

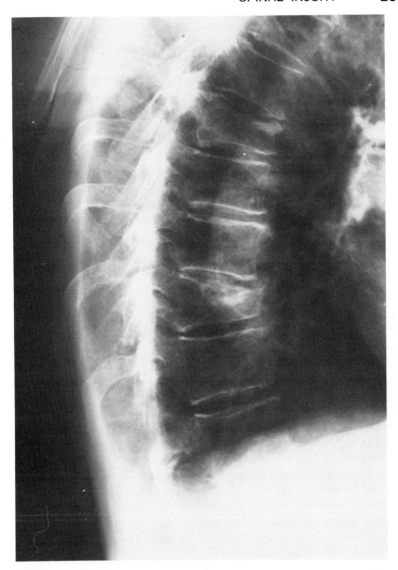

Figure 5.42.   Lateral roentgenogram of wedge compression fracture of thoracic vertebrae.

enough tensile stress to produce posterior ligament rupture. This injury does not produce acute instability and thus is not associated with neurological deficit. The fracture seldom involves the posterior cortex of the body, but, with comminution, fragments may protrude posteriorly and, in rare instances, produce neurological deficit.

Flexion Rotation

The *1st* to *10th* thoracic vertebrae articulate with the ribs in such a way as to increase resistance to torsion. The lumbar spine has a high torsional stiffness due in part to the orientation of the facet. However, the region between T10 and L1 has relatively great rotational mobility and therefore is susceptible to flexion rotation stress and fracture dislocation. The lesion is usually unstable and is associated with a high incidence of neurological deficit (60–70%).

Lateral Flexion

Excessive lateral bending produces asymmetrical loading of the vertebral body and may result in a lateral wedge fracture (Fig. 5.43). This fracture is relatively uncommon but when seen is usually in the lumbar spine.[35]

Extension

Hyperextension forces commonly cause cervical fractures, but these are rare in the thoracolumbar spine or lumbar regions. Because of its kyphosis and rigidity, the thoracic spine resists extension injury-producing forces.

LUMBAR SPINE

The lumbar spine has the same basic structure as the cervical and thoracic spines but has greater stability and resistance to stress than the cervical spine. The vertebral body is massive; the end plates are parallel and are connected by intervertebral discs and strong annular fibrosis which is supported anteriorly and posteriorly by longitudinal ligaments. The facets are large; the superior facet faces medially and posteriorly, while the inferior facet faces anterolaterally. The strong ligamentum flavum and interspinous and supraspinatus ligaments, which make up the "posterior ligament" complex, add to its stability. The curve is lordotic and the spinous processes limit extension.

The lumbar spine is subjected to the same forces as other regions of the spine, but the dominant force is flexion and flexion rotation, with extension and compression being less common as a cause of injury to the lumbar spine.

Flexion

When the dominant force is flexion, the posterior ligament complex remains intact; energy is dissipated at the fulcrum and produces a wedge compression fracture. The anterior portion of the body collapses in compression but the end plates are preserved. Radiologically, the alignment of the spinous processes is maintained and there is no widening or

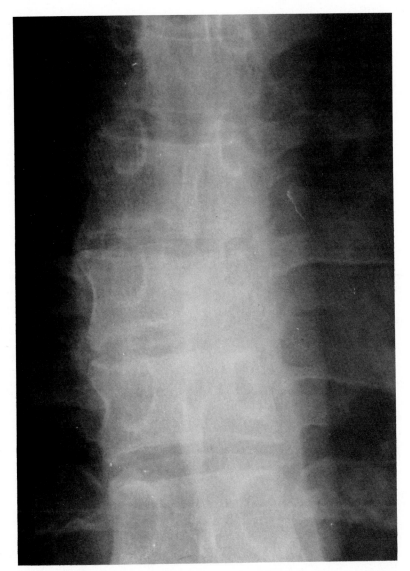

Figure 5.43. Lateral wedge compression of fracture of thoracic spine.

gap between the processes. The spine is stable and there is no associated neurological deficit.

Flexion Rotation

Where the rotation element is dominant, the posterior ligament complex is disrupted, allowing the energy to be expended through the capsular ligament and intervertebral disc or a portion of the vertebral body. This results in either a dislocation or fracture dislocation (Fig. 5.44).

Dislocation

This will result if the flexion component is sufficiently powerful to disengage the facets. Disruption through the posterior ligament complex, capsules, and intervertebral discs will produce dislocation with locking of the facets. This dislocation can occur at any level but is more common at the dorsolumbar junction. Radiologically, the spine will be in alignment, but a gap will be noted between the spinous processes at the level of the lesion (Fig. 5.45*A*) and will be palpable clinically (Fig. 5.45*B*). The lateral view will show the obvious dislocation and displacement (Fig. 5.45*C* and *D*).

Fracture Dislocation

Where the flexion component is insufficient to disengage the facets, and rotational force is dominant, the posterior ligament complex will rupture and the facets will fracture, producing a shearing of the superior plate or a wedge fracture of the vertebrae below. The lesion is very unstable, and may appear to reduce when the patient is supine.

Radiologically, the AP projection reveals the "telltale gap" (Fig. 5.46*A* and *B*) between the spinous processes and a malrotation which is palpable clinically (Fig. 5.46*C*). At the dorsolumber junction there may be a dislocation of the 12th rib on one side. Lateral projection reveals the

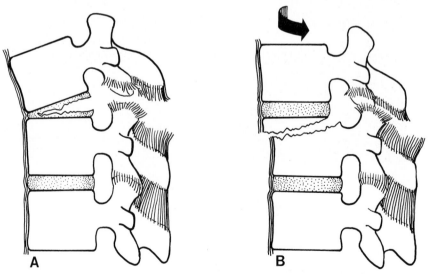

Figure 5.44.   *A*, ligamentous disruption secondary to flexion-rotation resulting in dislocation of the dorsolumbar spine. *B*, fracture dislocation.

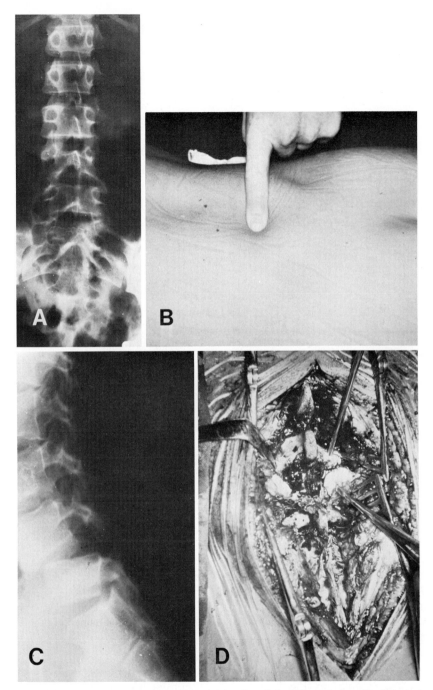

Figure 5.45. *A*, AP roentgenogram of L4–L5 dislocation of showing interspinous gap. *B*, clinical photograph of palpable interspinous gap. *C*, lateral roentgenogram of dislocation L4–L5 (locked facets). *D*, operative photograph of locked facets (L4–L5).

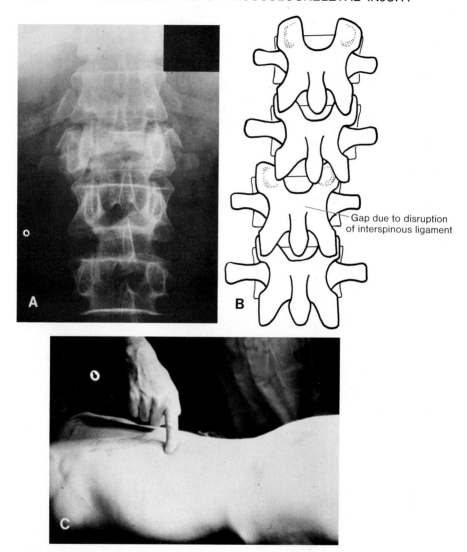

Figure 5.46.   An A, roentgenogram of fracture dislocation of T12-L1 showing interspinous gap and malalignment of spinous processes. B, drawing of interspinous gap and malalignment of spinous processes. C, clinical palpation of interspinous gap.

wedge slice fracture of the vertebral body, but this may not be obvious in the supine position (Fig. 5.47). The common location for this lesion is in the thoracolumbar junction, and there is a high incidence of neurological involvement.

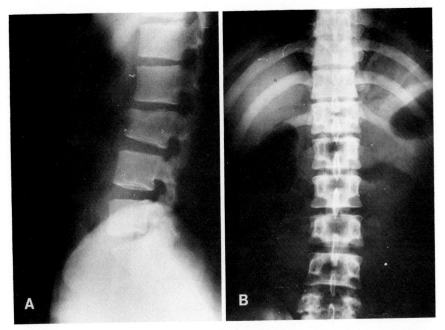

Figure 5.47.   Roentgenograms of *A*, lateral view of L2–L3 fracture dislocation with slice fracture vertebral body; lesion appears minimal in supine (reduced) position. *B*, AP of L2–L3 fracture dislocation; interspinous gap indicates instability.

At the T12-L1 junction the lesion may involve the cord or nerve roots or both.[17, 18] The spinal cord ends at the lower border of L1. The first sacral segment lies opposite the lower border of T12. The first lumbar segment lies opposite T9. All lumbar cord segments lie between T9 and T12. All sacral segments lie between T12 and L1 (Fig. 5.48). Thus, at T12 the vertebral canal contains all the lumbar nerve roots passing from the highest segments of origin to respective foramina of exit. Cord injury level is at the radiological level of the bony injury. Permanent cord transection will be signalled clinically by the presence of a glans bulbar and an anal reflex in the absence of sensation and motor power below the level of the cord lesion.[17, 18, 42] The level of neurological abnormality may be higher because of root involvement. The roots may be spared or contused and capable of recovery (Fig. 5.49*A*), or they may be transected (Fig. 5.49*B*). In the latter instance, the higher neurological deficit will be permanent. In the former, the patient may recover but have a lower level of deficit on final assessment. However, there may be a combination of root sparing, contusion, and transection (Fig. 5.49*C*). At this level, spinal

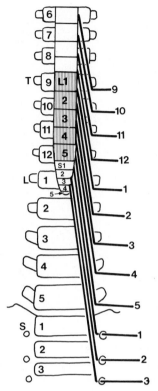

Figure 5.48.   Relationship of cord and nerve roots to vertebrae.

instability is hazardous and the cord and roots require protection through stabilization of the spine.

Extension

As a mechanism of injury in the lumbar spine, extension is less common than flexion for flexion rotation. There is no disruption of the anterior longitudinal ligament. Hyperextension causes impingement on the spinous processes and results in fracture of the spinous processes or lamina. This injury is not usually associated with neurological impairment.

Compression

As in the cervical spine, the lumbar vertebrae align in a vertical manner during flexion from the extended position (Fig. 5.50). Axial loading forces the incompressible nucleus pulposus against the end plate. Thereupon nuclear material is forced into the vertebral body in an explosive manner, producing a burst fracture of the body vertebrae[17] (Fig. 5.51). The

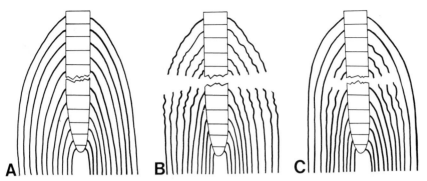

Figure 5.49.   *A,* cord transection, roots intact. *B,* cord and root transection. *C,* cord transection with some root involvement.

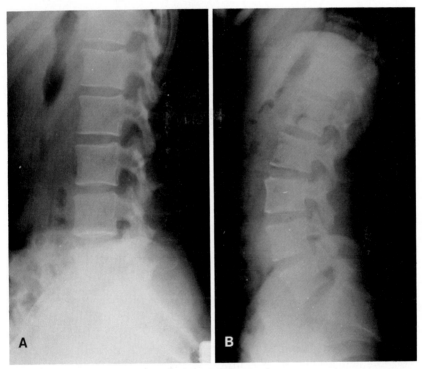

Figure 5.50.   *A,* Roentgenogram of lumbar vertebrae in vertical alignment. Compression in this position produces a brust fracture. *B,* normal lumbar lordosis.

posterior ligament complex remains intact and confers stability on the spine, in that there is no translation of the fragments. However, the comminuted body may become compressed and late localized kyphosis may develop. Neurological sparing is usual.

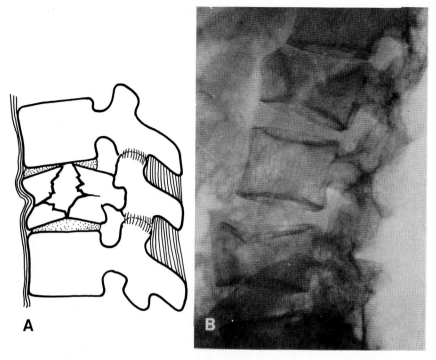

Figure 5.51. *A,* Burst fracture of the lumbar spine-vertebral body. *B,* lateral view (roentgenogram).

Distraction

Distraction injury occurs most commonly in the lumbar spine and is almost exclusively secondary to the lap seat belt in motor vehicle accidents. The lesion is described below under the heading "Lap Seat Belt Injury."

BIOMECHANICAL-CLINICAL CONSIDERATIONS

Lap Seatbelt Injury

A lap seatbelt acting as the restraining device in rapid deceleration motor vehicle accidents often produces a distraction injury with a characteristic fracture pattern. The lap belt acts as a fulcrum, impeding forward thrust of the lower trunk and pelvis, and the forces are focussed in the area of restraint.[39] The upper trunk, arms, and lower limbs, being unrestrained, shoot forward in a centrifugal manner, increasing the distraction force posteriorly in the lumbar spine (Fig. 5.52A). The section on biomechanics of the spinal unit pointed out that during hyperflexion, the anterior part of the vertebral body is subjected to a compression force that is four times greater than the tension force generated at the interspinous ligament (Fig. 5.52B); this force crushes the anterior part of the vertebral body before the interspinous ligament can disrupt.[33] However, when a seatbelt restrains the trunk and operates as a fulcrum, the flexion axis is shifted forward to the point of contact of the belt with the anterior abdominal wall (Fig. 5.52C). The entire spine is posterior to the flexion axis and all components are subjected to tension stress and exposed to pure distraction (tension) injury. The following fracture patterns occur:[39]

1. Pure ligamentous disruption, interspinous ligament, articular capsules, ligamentum flava, and posterior longitudinal ligament (Fig. 5.53A);
2. Ligamentous disruption with the avulsion of one or both articular processes (Fig. 5.53B);
3. Avulsion fracture of posterior inferior portion of the body of the vertebrae above (Fig. 5.53C).

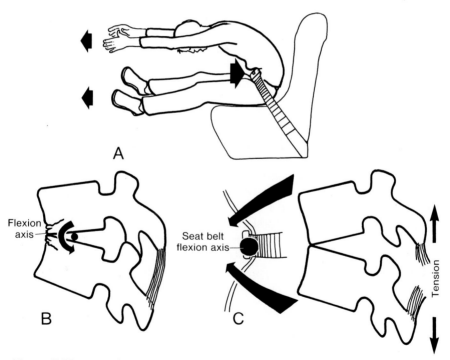

Figure 5.52. *A*, occupant of motor vehicle being thrust forward against seat belt. *B*, normal axis of spinal unit. *C*, axis of rotation shifts forwards to seat belt. The elements posterior to the seat belt are under distraction (tension).

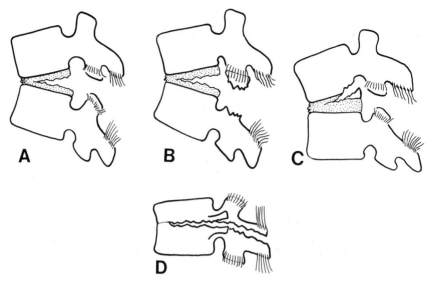

Figure 5.53. Ligamentous disruption due to distraction (*A*) and with articular process avulsion (*B*). *C*, Avulsion fracture of posterior portion of body. *D*, Chance fracture extends through body and spinous process.

4. Horizontal fracture extending across the vertebral body, pedicle, transverse process, lamina, and spinous process (Chance fracture)[4] (Fig. 5.53*D*).

It is to be noted that the absence of (or minimal) anterior compression of the vertebral body and the absence of translation (forward or lateral displacement) and no oblique fracture line indicate that there is little or no rotational or compression force component. Further, it has been observed that the distraction injury as described above seldom occurs in the driver of a motor vehicle. Presumably the steering wheel limits the forced flexion and forward thrust, thus decreasing the tension stress generated posteriorly. The lesion is more common in the passenger who suffers no limitation to the flexion which occurs over a seatbelt or edge of the top of the front seat. Because there is no lateral or anterior displacement or rotation disruption, it is unusual to encounter any neurological deficit.

THE KINETICS OF REAR-END COLLISION
(Acceleration-Deceleration or Whiplash Injury)

Whiplash injury of the cervical spine is due to *indirect trauma* from acceleration-deceleration (inertia) forces. The injuries are produced by inertia forces only, because the head and neck are usually not subjected to direct trauma.

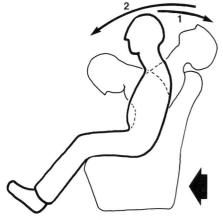

Figure 5.54 Motor vehicle occupant—movement sequence on rear end impact.

Inertia is that property of a body which resists any change in its position of rest or motion. Sudden deceleration of a vehicle causes the body to move forward relative to the seat. On the other hand, if the vehicle is accelerated, the body is pushed back against the seat. The magnitude of the force applied to the body, "inertia force," depends on the mass of the object and the rate of acceleration. The inertia force always acts in a direction opposite to that of acceleration, and is expressed by the equation $F = M \cdot a,$ where F is inertia force, m is the mass, and a is acceleration.

When a car is struck from the rear it moves forward; i.e., it is accelerated by the impact of the collision. The torso of a person sitting in the automobile is accelerated forwards with the vehicle, while the unrestrained head and neck lag behind owing to their "inertia." As illustrated in Figure 5.54, the inertia force acts to displace the head opposite to the direction of the car's acceleration. Since the mass of the head and neck is constant, the magnitude of the inertia force will depend almost entirely on the acceleration values. Using anthropometric dummies in a rear-end accident situation, Severy[38] has demonstrated the effect of impact on the vehicle.[22] A staged impact at 8 mph produced the typical acceleration time curve shown in Figure 5.55. The duration of impact, 200 msec, is relatively long, but the acceleration peak for the car is not particularly high. The acceleration curves for the shoulder and head illustrate that there is considerable lag in the system due to deformation of the body parts and deflection of the seat system. Indeed, peak accelerations for these structures occur at magnitudes significantly higher than those recorded for the vehicle. Severy concluded from these experiments that "whiplash injuries" produce rotational and translational accelerations larger than those of the vehicle itself.

The inertia force (Fig. 5.56A) will exert two different effects on the

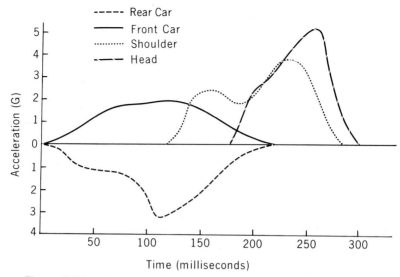

Figure 5.55.   Acceleration-time relationship from a staged collision.

neck. Because of translation, the initial movement of the head is rearward relative to the torso and produces a shearing type of displacement of the neck. The degree of bending due to the inertia force will depend on the value of "*d*" and will be maximum at the base of the spine, thus producing an extension strain. The individual with a long, thin neck is subject to greater force than one with a short, thick "bull" neck. The head is also subjected to high rotational acceleration (angular acceleration), during which the axis of rotation is located at the base of the skull and upper cervical region. This rotation effect will be transmitted to the cervical spine as an extension torque. In severe injuries the neck may extend until the occupant is facing the rear of the car (Fig. 5.56*B*). The neck may then, because of linear acceleration, be subjected to almost pure distraction (tension force).

Resistance to extension is initially provided by the anterior neck muscles. When the tone of the cervical muscles is overcome, there is nothing to resist the extension moment except the anterior longitudinal ligament and the disc annulus. When acceleration has stopped, the head rebounds forward (Fig. 5.54), in part because of impact with the seat, vehicle deceleration, and stretch-reflex-mediated contraction of the anterior neck muscles.

Animal experimentation[49] has shown that acceleration-extension strains of the neck can give rise to a wide spectrum of pathological lesions, including muscle tears, disc ruptures, tearing of the anterior longitudinal ligament, esophageal and vertebral artery stretching, and damage to the

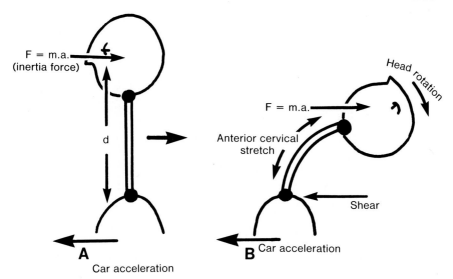

Figure 5.56. *A,* inertia force. *B,* inertia force: head in position of hyperextension before rebound.

cervical sympathetic chain. In addition, retro-ocular hematoma, middle ear and brain hemorrhage, and subdural hematoma have been observed. It is not possible to correlate these experimental findings with clinical experience because pathological data about these injuries in humans are scant. However, these experiments cast some light on the complaints of rear-end collision victims.

BIOMECHANICS OF SPINAL STABILIZATION

The spine is constructed of two subsystems, the compression-resisting anterior column and the tension-resisting posterior column.[7] A break in the multilinked column may produce immediate instability with a threat to nervous elements, or the spine may remain stable but be exposed to the possible development of late deformity and associated symptoms.

To be ideal, stabilization must restore and maintain the two columns and resist axial compression anteriorly, tension posteriorly, and rotation stress in all directions. The spine requires extrinsic mechanical stabilization until healing has restored the intrinsic stability. The biomechanics of the lesion and the region involved determines the method by which stability is restored.

Distraction rod application is a suitable method of stabilization in the unstable fracture dislocation produced by flexion rotation, in which the anterior longitudinal ligament is intact. Flexion rotation occurs most commonly in the dorsolumbar region and in the unsta-

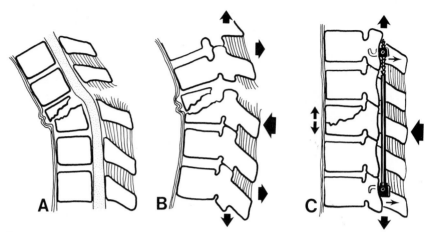

Figure 5.57. *A,* fracture dislocation of the dorsolumbar spine. *B,* distraction forces and three-point bending system. *C,* fracture reduction using distraction rods.

ble burst fracture[6, 11, 16] (Fig. 5.57*A*). Two distraction rods are placed posteriorly across the fracture and span two lamina above and below; they are fixed by means of hooks proximally and distally. The terminal distraction forces produce bending moments that tend to correct the deformity and are added to the forces of the three-point bending system[47] (Fig. 5.57*B*). The effect of the rods is to elongate the anterior column (which is limited by the intact anterior longitudinal ligament), to relieve the axial compression anteriorly, and to restore posterior stability (Fig. 5.57*C*).

Compression rods are applied to multiple compression fractures associated with intact posterior elements (flexion injury) (Fig. 5.58*A*). Usually these occur in a region characterized by a natural kyphosis (thoracic spine) or in the presence of a severe single compression fracture which produces a localized kyphosis.[11] These lesions may progress to produce late deformity. The rods are placed posteriorly with the hooks proximal and distal to the fracture. The effect is to produce a three-point bending system that provides a push at the center over the apex and a pull at the end, which tends to straighten the spine[47] (Fig. 5.58*B*). Anterior axial compression is reduced, preventing further deformity (Fig. 5.58*C*).

Compression Rods in Distraction Injuries

The distraction that develops from seat belt injuries results in ligamentous disruption or fracture through the body and posterior elements (Chance fracture).[4, 39] This lesion can readily be stabilized by restoring

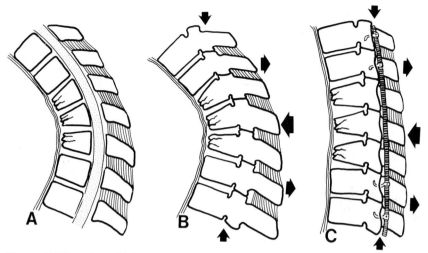

Figure 5.58. *A*, multiple compression fractures involving the thoracic spine. *B*, force application to reduce fracture. *C*, fracture reduction and compression rod stabilization.

tension resistance through the application of short compression rods spanning one vertebra above the lesion and one below[11, 48] (Fig. 5.59).

Stabilization in Flexion Rotation Fracture Dislocation of the Cervical Spine

Posterior Stabilization

The dislocation or fracture dislocation of the cervical spine which develops after flexion rotation is unstable and is characterized by disruption posteriorly, with compression fracture anteriorly or disc disruption but with an intact anterior longitudinal ligament (Fig. 5.60*A*). Stabilization is readily achieved by restoring tension resistance by the application of figure-of-eight wire or similar fixation between the spinous processes. This restores posterior stability (Fig. 5.60*B*).

Anterior Graft

Anterior interbody graft carried out in the presence of posterior instability breaches the anterior longitudinal ligament and may further interfere with the anterior column stability[24, 40] (Fig. 5.61*A* and *B*). With interference to both anterior and posterior columns, instability persists and thus renders the spine vulnerable to redisplacement (Fig. 5.61*C*).

In the management of spinal cord injury, the surgeon acts to prevent damage to nervous elements beyond that inflicted at the initial injury, to

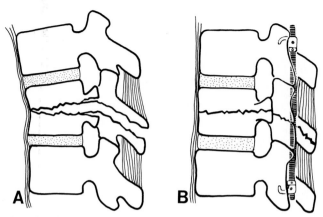

Figure 5.59.   *A,* chance fracture. *B,* fracture reduction and maintenance by means of short compression rods.

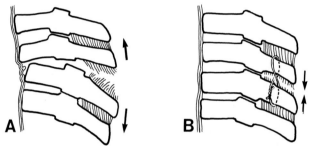

Figure 5.60.   *A,* fracture dislocation of the cervical spine. *B,* reduction and maintenance using interspinous wire fixation to restore tension resistance posteriorly.

preserve remaining function, to protect injured tissues and, finally, to provide optimum conditions for recovery. To achieve these objectives he requires an understanding of spinal biomechanics and must relate this to the mechanism of injury and to the pathology of resulting lesions. The mechanism of injury can be deduced by correlating clinical and radiological data with a knowledge of spinal lesions produced experimentally.

The effect of force applied to different regions of the spine depends on the anatomical characteristics of that region. There is a balance between stability and movement. In the production of spinal injury, forces (loads) act to produce deformation. The load varies according to *type* (bending, axial, torsion, tension, shear) *rate,* and *magnitude.* The deformation is resisted by the *material properties* (bone, ligaments, etc.) and *structural properties* (anatomical configuration) of the spine. In clinical assessment, loads are considered in terms of the movement they produce—flexion,

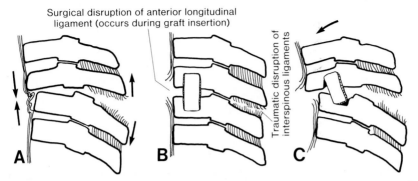

Figure 5.61. *A*, fracture dislocation of the cervical spine (flexion rotation). *B*, anterior interbody bone graft. *C*, redisplacement of fracture following anterior interbody graft. Instability is due to lack of posterior tension resistance restoration.

Table 5.2 Classification of Fractures of the Spine

Cervical Spine	
Atlantoaxial region	
Compression	Jefferson fracture
Flexion Rotation	1. Subluxation (rupture transverse ligament)
	2. Fracture odontoid
	3. Fracture dislocation C2–C3
Extension Rotation	1. Fracture arch C1–C2
	2. Fracture pedicle C2
	3. Traumatic spondylolisthesis of the axis
Cervical 3–7	
Compression	Burst fracture
Flexion Rotation	1. Subluxation
	2. Dislocation
	Unilateral locked facet
	Bilateral locked facet
	3. Fracture dislocation
	4. Compression fracture (flexion dominant)
Extension Rotation	1. Fracture dislocation
	2. Central cord syndrome
Thoracic Spine	
Flexion	Wedge compression fracture
Flexion Rotation	Fracture dislocation
Lateral Flexion	Lateral wedge fracture
Lumbar Spine	
Flexion	Compression fracture
Flexion Rotation	1. Dislocation
	2. Fracture dislocation
Extension	Fracture posterior elements
Compression	Burst fracture
Distraction	Chance fracture

extension, lateral bending, compression rotation, distraction, and translation. These movements usually occur in combination and seldom as single entities, although one or the other may be dominant. The effect of these loads or resultant movements are analyzed as if they applied to an isolated spinal unit (two linked vertebrae) in an experimental situation. The force pattern of compression, flexion rotation, extension rotation, and distraction is analyzed as it affects the multilinked vertebral column, comprising a compression-resisting anterior column and a tension-resisting posterior column in the clinical situation. Anatomical differences between the cervical, thoracic, and lumbar regions make it necessary to analyze separately the forces and resulting lesions in these three regions (see Table 5.2).

This chapter has discussed biomechanical factors as they relate to lap seatbelt injury and the kinetics of rear-end collision or accelerated-deceleration injury. The biomechanics of spinal stabilization are considered with particular reference to the application of distraction rods in fracture dislocation and compression rods in multiple compression fractures and in distraction injuries. It also emphasizes the importance of restoration of tension resistance in maintaining stability in fracture dislocation of the cervical spine and the vulnerability of an anterior interbody fusion in the presence of posterior instability.

References

1. BHALLA K, SIMMONS EH: Norman range of intervertebral joint motion of the cervical spine. *Can J Surg* 12:181–187, 1969.
2. BRASHEAR HR, VENETRS GC, PRESTON ET: Fractures of the neural arch of the axis. *J Bone Joint Surg* 57A:879–887, 1975.
3. BROWN T, HANSEN RJ, YORRA AJ: Some mechanical tests on the lumbosacral spine with particular reference to the intervertebral discs. *J Bone Joint Surg* 39A:1–135, 1957.
4. CHANCE GQ: Note on a type of flexion fracture of the spine. *Br J Radiol* 21:452–453, 1948.
5. DALL D: Personal communication.
6. DICKSON HH, HARRINGTON PR, ERWIN WD: Results of reduction and stabilization of the severely fractured thoracic and lumbar spine. *J Bone Joint Surg* 60A:799–805, 1978.
7. EVANS FG: Some basic aspects of biomechanics of the spine. *Arch Phys Med Rehab* 51:214–226, 1970.
8. FERLIC D: The range of motion of the "normal" cervical spine. *Bull Johns Hopkins Hosp* 110:59, 1962.
9. FIELDING JW, COCHRAN G van B, LANSING JF, MASON H: Tears of the transverse ligament of the atlas. *J Bone Joint Surg* 56A:1683–1691, 1974.
10. FIELDING JW, HAWKINS RJ: Roentgenographic diagnosis of the injured neck. *Am Acad Orthop Surg Inst Course Lect* 25:49–170, 1976.
11. FLESCH JR, LEIDER LL, ERICKSON DL, CHOU SN, BRADFORD DS: Harrington instrumentation and spine fusion for unstable fractures and fracture-dislocations of the thoracic and lumbar spine. *J Bone Joint Surg* 59A:143–153, 1977.

12. FRANCIS WR, FIELDING JW: Traumatic spondylolisthesis of the axis. *Orthop Clin North Am* 491:1011–1027, 1978.

13. FRAZER JE: *The Anatomy of the Human Skeleton* pp. 22–28. J & A Churchill, London, 1948.

14. GARBER JN: Abnormalities of the atlas and axis vertebrae—congenital and traumatic. *J Bone Joint Surg* 46A:1782–1791, 1964.

15. GRANT JCB: *An Atlas of Anatomy*, p. 273. Wiliam & Wilkins, Baltimore, 1948.

16. HARRINGTON PR, DICKSON JH: Reduction and stabilization: Treatment for the fractured spine using Harrington instrumentation. Zimmer USA Surgical Technique B-2254.

17. HOLDSWORTH FW: Fractures and dislocations of the lower thoracic and lumbar spines with and without neurological involvement. In *Current Practice in Orthopedic Surgery,* edited by JP Adams, vol. 2. CV Mosby, St. Louis, 1964.

18. HOLDSWORTH FW: Fractures, dislocations and fracture–dislocations of the spine. *J Bone Joint Surg* 45B:6–20, 1963.

19. JEFFERSON G: Fractures of the atlas vertebrae: report of four cases and review of those previously recorded. *Br J Surg* 7:407–421, 1920.

20. LUCAS DB: Mechanics of the spine. *Bull Hosp Joint Dis* 31:115–131, 1970.

21. MARKOLF KL: Deformation of the thoracolumbar intervertebral joints in response to external loads. *J Bone Joint Surg* 54A:511–533, 1972.

22. MARTINEZ JL, GARCIA DJ: A model for whiplash. *J Biomech* 1:23–32, 1968.

23. MORRIS JM: Biomechanics of the spine. *Arch Surg* 107:418–423, 1973.

24. MUNRO D: The factors that govern the stability of the spine. *Paraplegia* 3:219–228, 1966.

25. NACHEMSON AL, EVANS JH: Some mechanical properties of the third human lumbar interlaminar ligament ligamentum flavum. *J Biomech* 1:211–220, 1968.

26. ORNE D, LIU YK: A mathematical model of spinal response to impact. *J Biomech* 4: 49–71, 1971.

27. PANJABI MM, BRAND RA, WHITE AA: Three dimensional flexibility and stiffness properties of the human thoracic spine. *J Biomech* 9:185–192, 1976.

28. PANJABI MM, BRAND RA, WHITE AA: Mechanical properties of the human thoracic spine. *J Bone Joint Surg* 58A:642–651, 1976.

29. PANJABI MM, WHITE AA, JOHNSON RM: Cervical spine mechanics as a function of transection of components. *J Biomech* 8:327–336, 1975.

30. PENNAL G: Proceedings and reports of councils and associations. *J Bone Joint Surg* 48B:180, 1966.

31. PENNAL GF, McDONALD GA, DALE GA: Stress studies of the lumbar spine. *J Bone Joint Surg Br* 46B:786, 1966.

32. RAND RW, CRANDALL PH: Central spinal cord syndrome in hyperextension injuries of the cervical spine. *J Bone Joint Surg* 44A: 1415–1422, 1962.

33. ROAF R: A study of the mechanics of spinal injuries. *J Bone Joint Surg* 42B:810–823, 1960.

34. ROBERTS VL, NOYES FR, HUBBARD RP, McCABE J: Biomechanics of snowmobile spine injuries. *J Biomech* 4:569–577, 1971.

35. ROCKWOOD CA, GREEN DP: *Fractures,* vol. 2, pp. 873–884. JB Lippincott, Philadelphia, 1975.

36. SALDEEN T: Fatal neck injuries caused by use of diagonal safety belts. *J Trauma* 7: 856–862, 1967.

37. SCHNEIDER RC, CHERRY G, PANTEK H: The syndrome of acute central cervical spinal cord injury, with special reference to the mechanisms involved in hyperextension injuries of the cervical cord. *J Neurosurg* 11:546, 1954.

38. SEVERY DM: Controlled automobile rear-end collision, an investigation of related engineering and medical phenomena. *Can Services Med J* 11:727–759, 1955.
39. SMITH WS, KAUFER H: Patterns and mechanisms of lumbar injuries associated with lap seat belts. *J Bone Joint Surg* 51A:239–254, 1969.
40. STAUFFER ES, KELLY EG: Fracture-dislocations of the cervical spine. *J Bone Joint Surg* 59A:45–48, 1977.
41. VIRGIN WJ: Experimental investigations into the physical properties of the intervertebral disc. *J Bone Joint Surg* 33B:607–611, 1951.
42. WATSON-JONES R: Fractures and Joint Injuries, vol. 11. E & S Livingstone, London, 1955.
43. WEIR DC: Roentgenographic signs of cervical injury. *Clin Orthop* 109:9–17, 1975.
44. WHITE AA: Analysis of the mechanics of the thoracic spine in man. *Acta Orthop Scand (Suppl)* 127:86–88, 1969.
45. WHITE AA: Kinematics of the normal spine as related to scoliosis. *J Biomech* 4:405–411, 1971.
46. WHITE AA, HIRSCH C: The significance of the vertebral posterior elements in the mechanics of the thoracic spine. *Clin Orthop* 81:2–41, 1971.
47. WHITE AA, PANJABI MM, THOMAS CL: The clinical biomechanics of kyphotic deformities. *Clin Orthop* 128:8–17, 1977.
48. WHITESIDES TE: Traumatic kyphosis of the thoracolumbar spine. *Clin Orthop* 128:78–92, 1977.
49. WICKSTROOM JK: Acceleration-deceleration injuries of the cervical spine in animals. Proceedings 7th Stapp Conferences, pp 276–284, 1963.
50. WILLIAMS TB: Hangmans Fracture, *J Bone Joint Surg* 57B:82–88, 1975.
51. WOOD-JONES F: The Ideal Lesion Produced by Judicial Hanging. Lancet. pp 53, 1913.

Questions—Chapter 5

1. In considering forces acting on the spine, compression produces:
   a. bending
   b. axial loading
   c. tension
   d. shear

2. In the clinical situation loads are considered in terms of the movement they produce. In this context shear produces:
   a. compression
   b. distraction
   c. translation
   d. rotation

3. In the erect posture the line of gravity intersects:
   a. C7-T10-S2
   b. C5-T10-S1
   c. C1-T9-S3
   d. C7-T12-S4

4. The spine can be considered as a two-column system, the anterior column (vertebral bodies) is —— resisting and the posterior column (neural arch) is —— resisting:
   a. compression and tension
   b. bending and rotation
   c. tension and compression
   d. translation and tension

5. In the normal adult spine, the vertebral end plate was found to fracture under an experimental load of:
   a. 100 lb
   b. 250 lb
   c. 300 lb
   d. 500 lb

6. The breaking point of the posterior interspinous ligament under tension is in the region of:
   a. 200 lb
   b. 50 lb

    c. 275 lb
    d. 400 lb

7. The intervertebral disc, capsular and interspinous ligament of a spinal unit are most vulnerable to:
    a. compression
    b. distraction
    c. rotation
    d. bending

8. There is greater movement during extension than during flexion at only two levels in the cervical spine:
    a. C2-3 and C3-4
    b. C1-2 and C3-4
    c. C6-7 and C7-I1
    d. C4-5 and C5-6

9. The maximum range of intervertebral movement occurs at:
    a. C2-3
    b. C3-4
    c. C4-5
    d. C5-6

10. The Jefferson fracture is caused by:
    a. flexion
    b. extension
    c. rotation
    d. compression

11. In the normal spine, radiologically a gap of — mm between the odontoid and the anterior arch of the atlas is within normal limits:
    a. 1 mm
    b. 0 mm
    c. 3 mm
    d. 5 mm

12. The transverse ligament has probably ruptured if the gap between the odontoid and the anterior arch of the atlas is:
    a. 0–2 mm
    b. 1–3 mm
    c. 3–5 mm
    d. 1–2 mm

13. Hangman's fracture is caused by extension compression or extension distraction and involves:

a. odontoid
b. C4-5
c. C5-6
d. C2-3

14. In the cervical spine the Burst fracture is caused by:
    a. rotation
    b. extension
    c. distraction
    d. compression

15. In the cervical spine, subluxation at the C5-6 level can best
    be demonstrated by:
    a. stereoscopic technique
    b. X-ray in the supine position
    c. X-ray in flexion and extension
    d. tomography

16. In the hangman's fracture the odontoid is:
    a. not involved
    b. fractured at the base
    c. displaced posteriorly and impinges on the cord
    d. fractured in the apical region

17. The unilateral locked facet in the cervical region results in a
    forward shift of the vertebral body by:
    a. a full body width
    b. not displaced
    c. more than 50% of the body width
    d. less than 50% of the body width

18. The AP X-ray of the cervical unilateral locked facet shows:
    a. the spinous processes to be in alignment
    b. the spinous process of the involved vertebrae to be dis-
    placed to the side of the facet shift
    c. the spinous process of the involved vertebrae to be dis-
    placed to the opposite of the facet shift
    d. the spinous process to be fractured and displaced inferiorly

19. In the cervical bilateral locked facet the AP X-ray shows:
    a. the spinous processes to be offset above the level of dislo-
    cation
    b. the spinous processes to be offset below the level of dislo-
    cation
    c. the spinous processes to be in alignment but with a gap
    d. the spinous processes to be in alignment and without a gap

20. A dislocation at the C6-7 level may be missed because all the cervical vertebrae are not visualized on a lateral projection of the cervical spine. The lesion can be demonstrated by:

a. a gap between the spinous processes on the AP view of the spine

b. oblique views

c. stereoscopic views

d. lateral X-ray with the patient prone

Index